Fetal Echocardiog

A Q&A REVIEW FOR THE ARDMS EXAMINATION

Fetal Echocardiography

A Q&A REVIEW FOR THE ARDMS EXAMINATION

2nd Edition

2018

Nikki C. Stahl, RT(R)(M)(CT), RDMS, RVT
Sonographer in High-Risk Obstetrics and Fetal Echocardiography
PinnacleHealth Maternal Fetal Medicine
Harrisburg, Pennsylvania

Valrie Kunes, BA, AS(R)
Sonographer in High-Risk Obstetrics and Fetal Echocardiography
Middleburg, Pennsylvania

Bradley W. Robinson, MD, FACC
Associate Professor of Pediatrics
Sidney Kimmel Medical College at Thomas Jefferson University
Nemours Cardiac Center
A. I. DuPont Hospital for Children
Wilmington, Delaware

DAVIES
PUBLISHING

Davies Publishing, Inc.
32 South Raymond Avenue
Pasadena, California 91105-1961
Phone 626-792-3046
Facsimile 626-792-5308
e-mail info@daviespublishing.com
www.daviespublishing.com

Michael Davies, Publisher
Charlene Locke, Production Manager
Christina J. Moose, Editorial Director
Janet Heard, Operations Manager
Jim Baun, Illustration
Satori Design Group, Inc., Design

Printed and bound in the United States of America

ISBN 978-0-941022-95-8

Library of Congress Cataloging-in-Publication Data

Names: Stahl, Nikki C., author. | Kunes, Valrie, author. | Robinson, Bradley W., author.
Title: Fetal echocardiography review : a Q&A review for the ARDMS examination
/ Nikki C. Stahl, Valrie Kunes, Bradley W. Robinson.
Description: 2nd edition. | Pasadena, California : Davies Publishing, Inc., 2017. | Includes bibliographical references.
Identifiers: LCCN 2016032624 | ISBN 9780941022958 (alk. paper)
Subjects: | MESH: Fetal Heart—ultrasonography | Fetal Heart—anatomy & histology | Heart Defects, Congenital—ultrasonography | Echocardiography—methods | Ultrasonography, Prenatal—methods | Examination Questions
Classification: LCC RG628.3.E34 | NLM WQ 18.2 | DDC 618.3/2075430076—dc23
LC record available at https://lccn.loc.gov/2016032624

Preface to the 2nd Edition

THIS MOCK EXAM is a question/answer/reference review of fetal echocardiography for those RDMS and RDCS candidates who plan to take the ARDMS specialty examination in fetal echocardiography. Cardiology fellows and pediatric cardiologists who are learning fetal echocardiography will also find this book very helpful. It is designed as an adjunct to your regular study and as a means of helping you determine your strengths and weaknesses so that you can study more effectively. *Fetal Echocardiography Review, 2nd Edition* covers everything on the current ARDMS exam content outline, which you will find at the end of this book with cross-references to the questions in this mock exam.

Facts about *Fetal Echocardiography Review*:

▸ This mock exam covers the material on the ARDMS exam content outline in effect as of 2018. Readers are advised to check the ARDMS website, www.ardms.org, for the latest updates. This mock exam itself is continuously updated and revised as necessary.

▸ This mock exam focuses exclusively on the Fetal Echocardiography specialty exam to ensure thorough coverage of even the smallest subtopic on the exam. (For the Sonography Principles and Instrumentation exam, see *Ultrasound Physics Review: SPI Edition*, by Cindy Owen and James Zagzebski, available at www.DaviesPublishing.com.)

▸ We use the most current ARDMS content outline as a guideline for coverage. It is, in fact, our table of contents. At the same time, we provide on pages xiii–xv a cross-referenced list of contents by specific topics and subtopics. Why? The ARDMS exam content outline provides a generalized categorical overview together with very specific clinical tasks, but it can miss key intermediate topics you must know to pass your exam. Hence our subject-driven cross-references give you the best of both worlds and confirm that we do in fact cover everything you should know.

▸ This second edition of *Fetal Echocardiography Review* contains 475 questions—23% more than the first edition. Many of these are illustrated with images and schematics.

▸ Explanations are clear and conveniently referenced for fact-checking or further study.

▸ While otherwise in ARDMS exam format, this Davies mock exam makes deliberate and judicious use of multiple-choice items with five, not four, possible choices—thereby increasing both the difficulty of each question and the time needed to answer it. We also sprinkle in a few answer-choice variants (such as "A and B" and "not/except" items). The point? To give you an educational tool that will exercise those neural pathways in more than one direction. Registry candidates who master these items at an average rate of 1 minute apiece will be exceptionally well prepared for the actual exam.

▸ The ARDMS exams include new Advanced Item Type (AIT) questions that assess practical sonography instrumentation skills. For the Fetal Echocardiography exam, these AIT questions include what ARDMS calls "Hotspot" questions. Hotspot items display an image and question, requiring you to indicate the correct answer by marking directly on the image using your cursor; this type of question is called "advanced" because it requires a higher level of thinking and processing than you perform when answering a conventional multiple-choice question. In Davies' mock exam, similar questions are identified as "AIT—Hotspot" questions. These items ask you to identify what an arrow in the image is pointing at or to indicate the label on an image that corresponds to the correct answer. Another type of AIT question, the "AIT—SIC" (Semi-Interactive Console)

item, requires the examinee to use a semi-interactive console to correct a problem with the image presented. These items are currently limited to the Sonography Principles and Instrumentation (SPI) examination, but as a bonus feature we have identified such items as "AIT—SIC" questions. Finally, PACSim items—case-based Picture Archive and Communication Simulation questions—are not included in the Fetal Echo mock exam because this type of question is specifically designed for and limited to physicians taking the Physician in Vascular Interpretation (PVI) exam.

▸ The expanded ARDMS exam content outline, complete with *all* questions that apply to specific clinical tasks, appears on pages 186–190. We have cross-referenced each task to the relevant question numbers in this Fetal Echo mock exam for your convenience in targeting your study on specific tasks. For the latest information on the Fetal Echo examination, please visit the ARDMS website at www.ardms.org.

Fetal Echocardiography Review effectively simulates the content of the exam. Current ARDMS standards call for 150 multiple-choice questions to be answered during a three-hour period. That is, you will have an average time of just over 1 minute to answer each question. Timing your practice sessions according to the number of questions you need to finish will help you prepare for the pressure experienced by Fetal Echo candidates taking this exam. It also helps to ensure that your practice scores accurately reflect your strengths and weaknesses so that you can study more efficiently in the limited time you are able to devote to preparation.

IMPORTANT NOTE: *Although many of our customers remark on similarities between our questions and those of the actual exam, do not be misled into thinking you should memorize these questions and answers. They are here to give you practice, to teach you things you may not know, and to reveal your strengths and weaknesses so that you know where to put your energy as you prepare for the exam.*

ARDMS test results are reported as a "scaled" score that ranges from a minimum of 300 to a maximum of 700. A scaled score of 555 is the passing score—the "passpoint" or "cutoff score" for all ARDMS examinations. The scaled score is simply a conversion of the number of correct answers that also, in part, takes into account the difficulty of a particular question. You can search on the Internet for *Angoff scoring method* if you want to learn more about scaled scoring. Suffice it to say that it helps to ensure the fairness of the exams. We include below and strongly recommend that you read *Taking and Passing Your Exam*, by Don Ridgway, RVT, who offers useful tips and practical strategies for taking and passing the ARDMS examinations.

Finally, you have not only our best wishes for success but also our admiration for taking this big and important step in your career.

Nikki C. Stahl

Valrie Kunes

Bradley W. Robinson

Nikki C. Stahl, RT(R)(M)(CT), RDMS, RVT
Valrie Kunes, BA, AS(R)
Bradley W. Robinson, MD, FACC

Taking and Passing Your Exam

by Don Ridgway, RVT*

Preparing for Your Exam . . .

Study. And then study some more. Knowing your stuff is the most important factor in your success. Start early, set a regular study schedule, and stick to it. Make your schedule specific so you know exactly what to study on a particular day. Write it down. Establish realistic goals so that you don't build a mountain you can't climb.

As to *what* you study, don't just read aimlessly. Focus your efforts on what you need to know. Rely on a core group of dependable references, referring to others as necessary to firm up your understanding of specific topics. Let the ARDMS exam outline guide you. And use different but complementary study methods—texts, flashcards, and mock exams—to exercise those neural pathways.

Ease down on studying the week before. Wind down, reduce stress, build confidence, and rest up. Don't cram! And no studying the night before. You had your chance. Watch a movie, relax, go to bed early, and sleep well.

Organize your things the night before. Lay out comfortable clothes (including a sweater or sweatshirt in case the testing center is cold), pencils, your ARDMS test-admission papers, car and house keys, glasses, prescriptions, directions to the test center, and any other personal items you might need. Be prepared!

The Day of Your Exam . . .

Eat lightly. You do not want to fall asleep during the exam. Go easy on the coffee or tea so your bladder doesn't distract you halfway through the exam.

Arrive early. Plan to arrive at the test center early, especially if you haven't been there before. Take directions, including the telephone number of the testing center in case you have to make contact en route. You don't need a wrong-offramp adventure.

Be confident. As you wait for the exam to begin, smile, lift both hands, wave them toward yourself, and say, "Bring it on."

During the Exam . . .

Read each question twice before answering. Guess how easy it is to get one word wrong and misunderstand the whole question!

Try to answer the question before looking at the choices. Formulating an answer before peeking at the possibilities minimizes the distractibility of the incorrect answer choices, which in the test-making business are called—guess what?—*distractors*.

---

*Don Ridgway is the author of *Introduction to Vascular Scanning: A Guide for the Complete Beginner* and editor of *Vascular Technology Review*. He is Professor Emeritus at Grossmont College in El Cajon, California.

Knock off the easy ones first. First answer the questions you feel good about. Then go back for the more difficult items. Next, attack the really tough ones. Taking notes on long or tricky questions often can jog your memory or put the question in new light. For questions you just cannot answer with certainty, eliminate the obviously wrong answer choices and then guess.

Guessing. Passing the exam depends on the number of correct answers you make. Because unanswered questions are counted as incorrect, it makes sense to guess when all else fails. The ARDMS itself advises that it is to the candidate's advantage to answer all possible questions. Guessing alone improves your chances of scoring a point from 0 (for an unanswered question) to 25% (for randomly picking one of four possible answers). Eliminating answer choices you know or suspect are wrong further improves your odds of success. By using your knowledge and skill to eliminate two of the four answer choices before guessing, for example, you increase your odds of scoring a point to 50%.

Pace yourself; watch the time. Work methodically and quickly to answer those you know, and make your best guesses at the gnarly ones. Leave no question unanswered.

Don't despair 50 minutes into the exam. At some point you may feel that things just aren't going well. Take 10 seconds to breathe deeply—in for a count of five, out for a count of five. Relax. Recall that you need only about three out of four correct answers to pass. If you've prepared reasonably well, a passing score is attainable even if you feel sweat running down your back.

Taking the Exam on Computer . . .

Some candidates express concern about taking the registry exam on a computer. Most folks find this to be pretty easy; some find it offputting, at least in prospect. But the computerized exams are quite convenient: You can take the exam at your convenience (a far cry from the days of one exam per year), you know whether or not you passed before you leave the testing center (compare that to waiting weeks and even months, as used to be the case), and you can reschedule the exam after 90 days if you happen not to pass the first time (rather than waiting another six months to a year). Another good point: The illustrations are said to be clearer on computer than in the booklets at a Scantron-type exam.

Taking the test by computer is not complicated. The center even gives you a tutorial to be sure you know what you need to do. You sit in a carrel with a computer and answer the multiple-choice questions by pointing and clicking with a mouse. There is a clock on the display letting you know how much time is left. Use it to pace yourself. Scratch paper is available; make liberal use of it.

You can mark questions for answering later. A display shows which questions have not been answered so you can return to them. When you have finished, you click on "DONE," and you find out immediately whether you passed.

It's nothing to be afraid of. The principles are the same as those for any exam. Be methodical and keep breathing.

Summary . . .

Preparing for the exam:

- Study.
- Use flashcards.
- Join a study group.
- Wind down a week before.
- Don't cram.
- Relax!

The day of your exam:

- Eat lightly, avoid coffee.
- Arrive early.
- Take a sweater.
- Be confident!

During the exam:

- Read each question twice.
- Answer the question before looking at the answer choices.
- Answer the easy ones first.
- Guess when necessary.
- Pace yourself.
- Don't despair.

Taking the exam on computer:

- Just point and click.
- Take notes.
- Mark and return to the hard questions.
- Use the on-screen clock to pace yourself.
- Be methodical.
- Breathe!

Contents

Contents by Subject Category

For your convenience, the questions in this mock exam are arranged here by subject.

Embryology

▸ timing of heart formation

▸ teratogenic insults

▸ atrial septal components

▸ endocardial cushion, d- and l-looping)

Indications

▸ maternal

▸ fetal

▸ environmental

Incidence of Congenital Heart Disease

▸ general population

▸ heredity

▸ chromosomal

▸ syndromes

▸ extracardiac anomalies

Timing of the Fetal Echocardiographic Exam

Standard Sonographic Views

▸ position/situs

▸ two-dimensional heart views

▸ Doppler hemodynamics

▸ M-mode

Normal Fetal Heart Anatomy

See questions 1, 2, 3, 8, 9, 10, 11, 12, 13, 26, 29, 30, 31, 36, 37, 39, 40, 44, 46, 50, 58, 61, 62, 71, 81, 377, 378, 379, 387, 389, 401.

▸ size

▸ venous connections

▸ atria and septum

▸ atrioventricular valves

▸ ventricles and septum

▸ outflow tracts

▸ semilunar valves

▸ great arteries

▸ pericardium

▸ other

Normal Fetal Heart Physiology

See questions 27, 45, 72, 75, 76, 77, 78, 79, 80, 82, 83, 84, 85, 86, 87, 88, 89, 90, 108, 128, 157, 174, 175, 176, 177, 178, 179, 180, 451, 452, 463, 466.

▸ heart rate

▸ blood flow and cardiac output

▸ in utero shunts

▸ series circulation

▸ structural heart anomalies

Structural Heart Anomalies

See questions 109, 110, 111, 113, 115, 116, 117, 129, 130, 132, 134, 135, 136, 137, 138, 139, 140, 141, 142, 143, 144, 145, 149, 150, 151, 152, 154, 158, 159, 160, 161, 162, 163, 164, 165, 166, 167, 168, 169, 170, 171, 172, 181, 182, 183, 184, 185, 186, 187, 188, 189, 190, 191, 192, 193, 194, 195, 196, 197, 198, 199, 200, 201, 202, 203, 204, 205, 206, 207, 208, 209, 210, 211, 212, 213, 214, 215, 216, 217, 218, 219, 220, 221, 222, 223, 224, 225, 226, 227, 228, 229, 230, 231, 232, 233, 234, 235, 236, 237, 238, 239, 240, 241, 242, 243, 244, 245, 246, 247, 248, 249, 250, 251, 252, 253, 254, 255, 256, 257, 258, 259, 260, 261, 262, 263, 265, 266, 267, 268, 269, 271, 272, 273, 274, 275, 276, 277, 278, 279, 280, 281, 282, 283, 306, 324, 327, 336, 341, 354, 359, 361, 362, 384, 402, 403, 467, 468, 469.

▸ cardiac malposition

▸ enlarged heart

▸ venous abnormalities

▸ atria and septum

▸ atrioventricular valves

▸ ventricles and septum

▸ semilunar valves

‣ great arteries

‣ pericardium

‣ complex cardiac anomalies

Dysrhythmias

See questions 105, 118, 119, 120, 121, 122, 123, 124, 125, 126, 127, 131, 320, 329, 334, 345, 390, 391, 397, 398, 470, 471, 472.

‣ bradyarrhythmias

‣ tachyarrhythmias

‣ ectopy

Acquired Pathology

See questions 112, 328, 331, 333, 335, 337, 338, 339, 342, 344, 473.

‣ metabolic/endocrine

‣ infection

‣ twin-to-twin transfusion

‣ intrauterine growth restriction

‣ drugs

Miscellaneous Pathology

See questions 48, 51, 106, 153, 264, 270, 284, 285, 286, 287, 288, 289, 290, 291, 292, 293, 294, 325, 351, 357, 453, 474.

‣ hydrops fetalis

‣ extracardiac anomalies

‣ syndromes

Physical Principles and Instrumentation

See questions 355, 356, 358, 392, 393, 394, 396, 404, 405, 406, 407, 408, 409, 410, 411, 412, 413, 414, 415, 416, 417, 418, 419, 420, 421, 422, 423, 424, 425, 426, 427, 428, 429, 430, 431, 432, 433, 434, 435, 436, 437, 438, 439, 440, 441, 442, 443, 444, 445, 446, 447, 448, 449, 450, 454, 455, 456, 457, 458, 459, 460, 461.

Patient Care

See questions 295, 296, 297, 298, 299, 300, 301, 464, 465, 475.

Color Plates

We have included this section of color flow images and spectral tracings to enhance the black-and-white versions used with some of the questions and answers in this mock exam. These images go with the questions referenced below, and they are cross-referenced from those questions to the color versions of the images that appear here. Each caption explains the image in relation to the question posed in the mock exam. For fuller information, we encourage you to refer to the image in the context of its question as well as its corresponding answer in Part 8, "Answers, Explanations, and References."

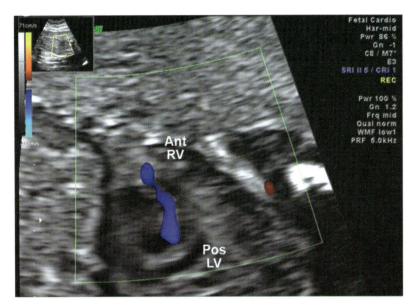

Color Plate 1 (page 34, question 170, and page 125, answer 170): This image is a short-axis view of the ventricles. The muscular septum is demonstrated at this level. Blood flow is seen shunting across the septum. This is abnormal and is diagnosed as a muscular ventricular septal defect.

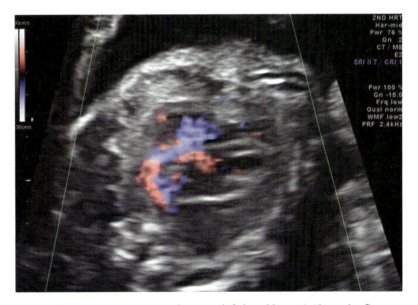

Color Plate 2 (page 49, question 247, left-hand image): The color flow demonstrated in this image could suggest a ventricular septal defect, overriding aorta, truncus arteriosus, and/or tetralogy of Fallot, but *not* a secundum atrial septal defect.

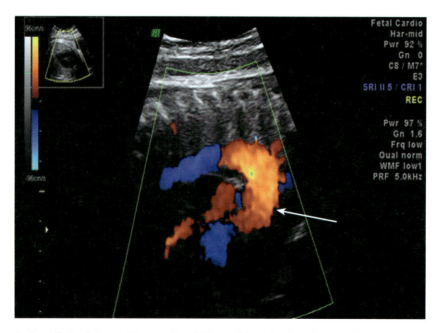

Color Plate 3 (page 78, question 372): In this color flow image, the arrow is pointing to the aortic arch.

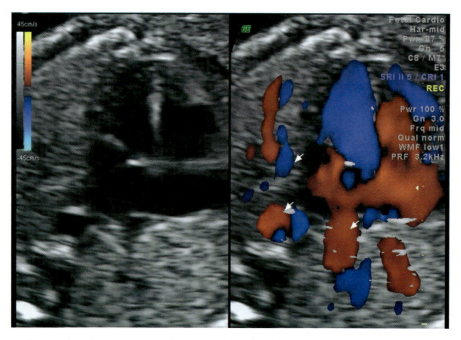

Color Plate 4 (page 80, question 380): The color flow image on the right demonstrates blood flow in the fetal pulmonary veins (arrows).

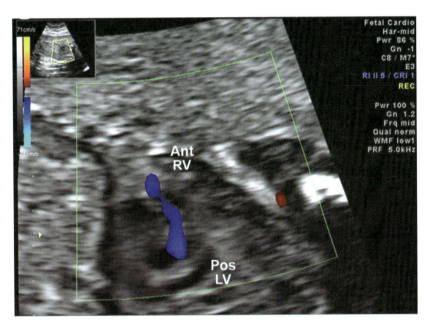

Color Plate 5 (page 81, question 384): This image is a short-axis view of the ventricles.

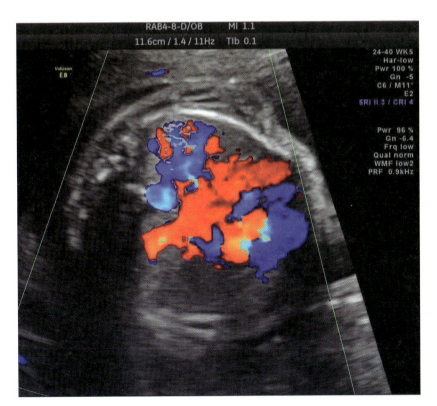

Color Plate 6 (page 93, question 419): To improve this image of a fetus in vertex presentation, pulse repetition frequency (PRF) should be increased. Increasing the PRF will decrease the number of pulses transmitted per second, eliminating the noise and scatter of the ultrasound frequencies.

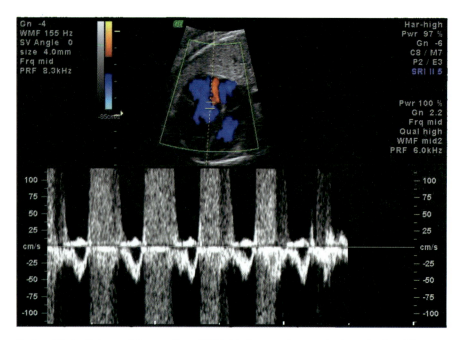

Color Plate 7 (page 96, question 432): This image demonstrates aliasing. The waveform has exceeded the maximum frequency available, therefore reaching the Nyquist limit. When the Nyquist limit is exceeded, the result is an aliasing artifact—due to the maximum Doppler frequency being reflected in the opposite direction.

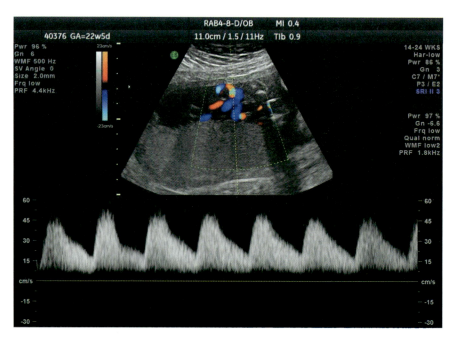

Color Plate 8 (page 97, question 434): In this Doppler tracing of the umbilical artery, the waveform does not completely fill the envelope. The low-level echoes near the baseline have been rejected and only the high-frequency echoes are displayed. Note the absence of signal near the baseline. For this image the wall filter was set too high.

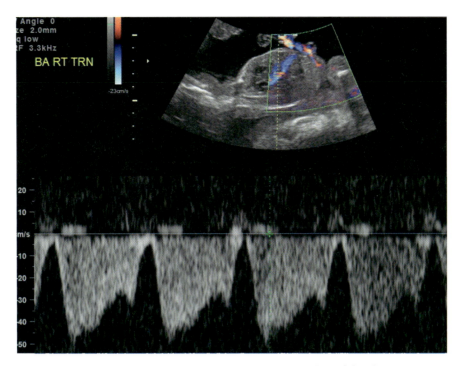

Color Plate 9 (page 97, question 435): This spectral tracing of the ductus venosus can be improved by decreasing the color gain.

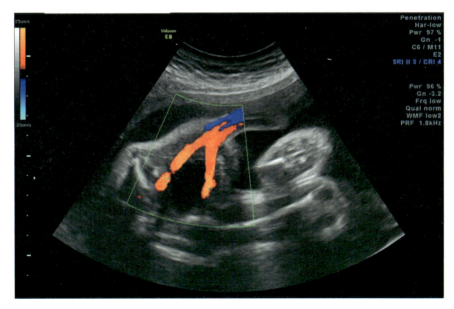

Color Plate 10 (page 99, question 438): This image was obtained using color Doppler imaging (also called *color flow imaging*), which displays blood flow velocity and direction (or other tissue motion) by assigning color to frequency-shifted echoes.

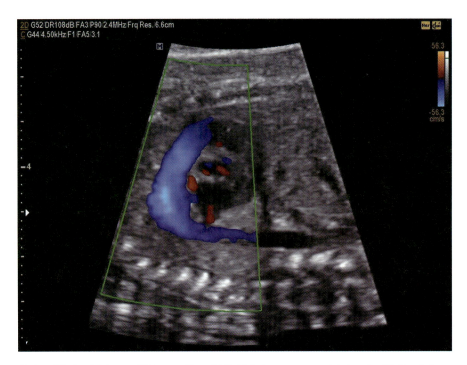

Color Plate 11 (page 100, question 441): This image was obtained with the fetus in breech presentation, head to maternal right and spine down. The color Doppler spectrum demonstrates both antegrade flow and continuous flow. The flow across the ductus arteriosus is a continuous forward, antegrade flow without any signs of reversal/retrograde flow. The color box shows the flow leaving the right ventricle and flowing away from the transducer in the normal antegrade fashion.

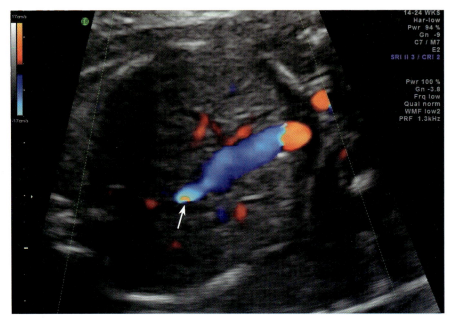

Color Plate 12 (page 100, question 442): The arrow in this image is pointing to the ductus venosus. The variation in the color signal in this image is due to aliasing.

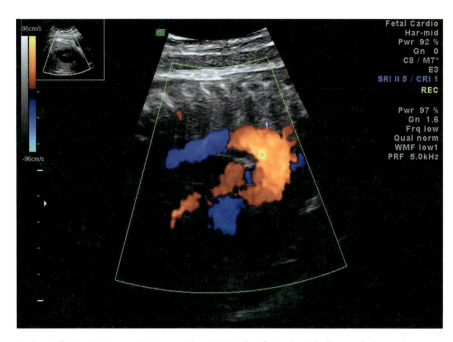

Color Plate 13 (page 101, question 443): The fetus in this image is in vertex presentation, spine up. The color spectrum demonstrates antegrade flow across the aortic arch.

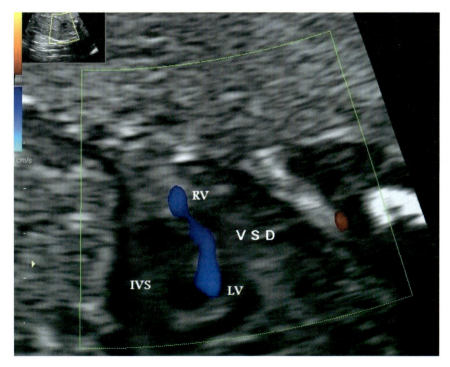

Color Plate 14 (page 101, question 445): A large muscular ventricular septal defect is seen in this image. The flow across the defect is from the right ventricle to the left ventricle.

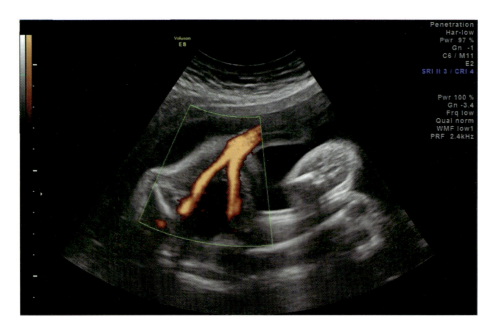

Color Plate 15 (page 102, question 447): Power Doppler was used to obtain this image. This mode (also known as *Doppler-power display* or *color power Doppler*) overcomes some of the limitations of conventional color Doppler imaging, and is valuable in detecting flow in low-flow states, producing better edge definition and depiction of continuity of flow when optimal Doppler angles cannot be obtained. Power Doppler is a "nondirectional" flow Doppler, as opposed to "directional-dependent flow" with standard color Doppler.

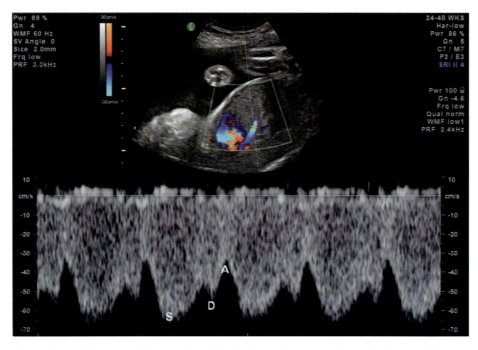

Color Plate 16 (page 104, question 455): In this pulsed-wave Doppler signal of the ductus venosus, the waveform demonstrates triphasic flow.

PART 1

Anatomy and Physiology

Normal anatomy and physiology

Evaluate aortic arch

Evaluate cardiac chambers

Evaluate cardiac septa and related structures

Evaluate cardiac valves

Evaluate coronary vessels

Evaluate ductal arch

Evaluate fetal anatomic structures related to the abdomen/pelvis

Evaluate fetal anatomic structures related to the chest/thorax

Evaluate fetus for normal cardiac axis, cardiac position, and abdominal situs

Evaluate pulmonary vessels

Evaluate systemic vessels

Evaluate tissues composing the heart

Perfusion and function

Evaluate for normal cardiac rhythms

Evaluate for normal fetal circulation

Organ development

Assess for normal embryologic development

Perform various fetal echocardiographic examinations during appropriate time intervals

1. What is the most superior structure in the fetal heart?
   A. Aorta
   B. Mitral valve
   C. Tricuspid valve
   D. Main pulmonary artery
   E. Superior vena cava

2. Approximately how large is the isthmus of the aorta in relation to the ascending and descending aorta?
   A. The same size
   B. 1/3 larger
   C. 1/3 the diameter
   D. 2/3 larger
   E. 2/3 smaller

3. Which of the following is TRUE about the normal left aortic arch?
   A. It gives off an innominate branch coursing to the right.
   B. It gives off the innominate artery, which divides into two branches.
   C. It gives off the brachiocephalic artery, which divides into the right subclavian and right common carotid arteries.
   D. It curves over the right pulmonary artery.
   E. All of the above are true.

Questions 4–7 refer to the following long-axis view of the fetal aortic arch.

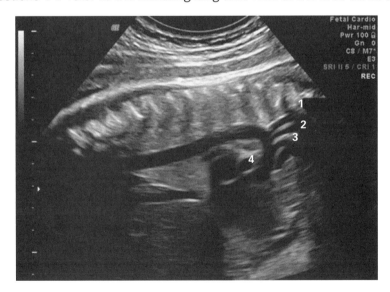

4. Number 1 represents the:
   A. Innominate artery
   B. Left common carotid artery
   C. Left subclavian artery

    D. Right pulmonary artery

    E. Superior vena cava

AIT—Hotspot item.*

5. Number 2 represents the:
    A. Innominate artery
    B. Left common carotid artery
    C. Left subclavian artery
    D. Right pulmonary artery
    E. Superior vena cava

AIT—Hotspot item.

6. Number 3 represents the:
    A. Innominate artery
    B. Left common carotid artery
    C. Left subclavian artery
    D. Right pulmonary artery
    E. Superior vena cava

AIT—Hotspot item.

7. Number 4 represents the:
    A. Right atrium
    B. Left atrium
    C. Superior vena cava
    D. Right pulmonary artery
    E. Persistent left superior vena cava

AIT—Hotspot item.

8. The most anterior structure of the normal fetal heart is the:
    A. Right atrium
    B. Right ventricle
    C. Pulmonary artery
    D. Left ventricle
    E. Aorta

9. The moderator band is the morphologic marker for the:
    A. Left ventricle
    B. Left atrium
    C. Right ventricle
    D. Right atrium
    E. Interventricular septum

---

*Advanced Item Type (AIT) Hotspot items marked here are similar to Hotspot items on the ARDMS exam. On the exam, these Hotspot items require you to indicate the correct answer by marking directly on the image using your cursor. In Davies' Fetal Echo mock exam, similar questions are identified as **AIT—Hotspot** and ask you to identify what an arrow in the image is pointing at or to indicate the label on an image that corresponds to the correct answer. Another type of AIT question, the **AIT—SIC** (Semi-Interactive Console) item, requires you to use a semi-interactive console to correct a problem with the image presented. These items are limited to the Sonography Principles and Instrumentation (SPI) examination, but as a bonus feature we have also identified these items in the Fetal Echo mock exam.

10. Which of the following is NOT true of the normal left atrium?
    A. It accepts the pulmonary veins.
    B. It contains the mitral valve.
    C. It accepts the foramen ovale flap.
    D. It is the chamber closest to the fetal spine.
    E. It is the most posterior heart chamber.

11. Which of the following are characteristics of the left ventricle?
    A. Septophobic mitral valve with attachments away from the septum
    B. Smooth walls
    C. Two papillary muscles
    D. Mitral valve more superior than tricuspid valve
    E. All of the above

12. Which of the following characterizes the left atrium?
    A. It has a finger-like, thin appendage.
    B. It receives the superior and inferior venae cavae.
    C. It has a broad-based appendage.
    D. It contains the sinoatrial node.
    E. All of the above.

13. The normal right ventricle:
    A. Has a moderator band
    B. Is very trabeculated
    C. Has a septophilic tricuspid valve with attachments to the septum
    D. Is triangular
    E. Exhibits all of these characteristics

Questions 14–16 refer to the following image of a normal fetal heart with {S, D, S} and normally related great vessels. The fetus is in the vertex presentation.

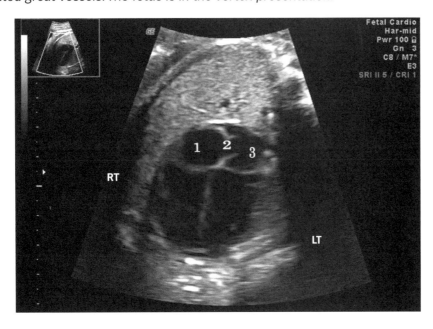

14. Number 1 represents the:
    A. Left atrium
    B. Right atrium
    C. Foramen ovale
    D. Coronary sinus
    E. Pulmonary veins

AIT—Hotspot item.

15. Number 2 represents the:
    A. Left atrium
    B. Right atrium
    C. Foramen ovale
    D. Coronary sinus
    E. Pulmonary veins

AIT—Hotspot item.

16. Number 3 represents the:
    A. Left atrium
    B. Right atrium
    C. Foramen ovale
    D. Coronary sinus
    E. Pulmonary veins

AIT—Hotspot item.

Questions 17–25 refer to the following image of a fetus in a vertex presentation, spine down, with a normal heart anatomy {S, D, S}.

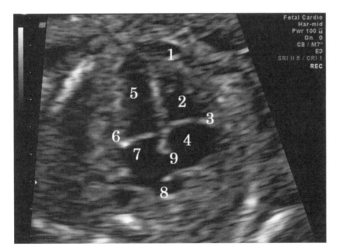

17. Number 1 represents the:
    A. Left ventricle
    B. Right ventricle
    C. Moderator band
    D. Foramen ovale
    E. Pulmonary veins

AIT—Hotspot item.

18. Number 2 represents the:
    A. Right ventricle
    B. Left ventricle
    C. Tricuspid valve
    D. Mitral valve
    E. Moderator band
AIT—Hotspot item.

19. Number 3 represents the:
    A. Right ventricle
    B. Left ventricle
    C. Tricuspid valve
    D. Mitral valve
    E. Moderator band
AIT—Hotspot item.

20. Number 4 represents the:
    A. Left ventricle
    B. Right ventricle
    C. Left atrium
    D. Right atrium
    E. Coronary sinus
AIT—Hotspot item.

21. Number 5 represents the:
    A. Right ventricle
    B. Left ventricle
    C. Tricuspid valve
    D. Mitral valve
    E. Moderator band
AIT—Hotspot item.

22. Number 6 represents the:
    A. Right ventricle
    B. Left ventricle
    C. Tricuspid valve
    D. Mitral valve
    E. Moderator band
AIT—Hotspot item.

23. Number 7 represents the:
    A. Left ventricle
    B. Right ventricle
    C. Left atrium
    D. Right atrium
    E. Coronary sinus
AIT—Hotspot item.

24. Number 8 represents the:
    A. Right atrium
    B. Left atrium
    C. Coronary sinus
    D. Foramen ovale
    E. Pulmonary veins

AIT—Hotspot item.

25. Number 9 represents the:
    A. Right atrium
    B. Left atrium
    C. Coronary sinus
    D. Foramen ovale
    E. Pulmonary veins

AIT—Hotspot item.

26. Which of the following statements about evaluating the interventricular septum is TRUE?
    A. Ventricular wall thickness should be measured in the subcostal four-chamber view.
    B. Ventricular wall thickness remains less than 5 mm throughout gestation.
    C. Ventricular septal wall thickness should be measured at end diastole.
    D. Both A and B are true statements.
    E. All of these statements are true.

27. Which of the following would be considered a normal fetal heart shunt?
    A. Ductus venosus
    B. Ductus arteriosus
    C. Patent foramen ovale
    D. B and C
    E. A, B, and C

28. The fetus in this image is in the vertex presentation with the fetal spine down. The heart has {S, D, S} relationship with normally related great arteries. The cardiac structure being measured is the:

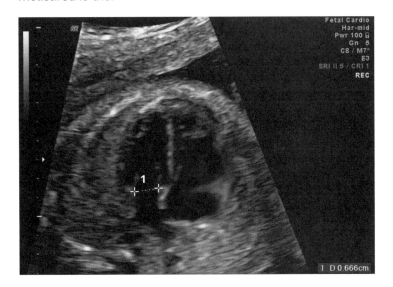

    A. Mitral valve

    B. Tricuspid valve

    C. Left atrium

    D. Right atrium

    E. Coronary sinus

AIT—Hotspot item.

29. The normal aortic valve consists of:
    A. 1 cusp
    B. 2 cusps
    C. 3 cusps
    D. 4 cusps
    E. 5 cusps

30. The normal mitral valve:
    A. Is attached more apically than the tricuspid leaflets
    B. Is continuous with the posterior wall of the aorta
    C. Has anterior, posterior, and septal leaflets
    D. Both A and C
    E. All of the above

31. What is the normal relationship of the semilunar valves?
    A. The aortic valve is to the right and posterior to the pulmonic valve.
    B. The aortic valve is to the right and anterior to the pulmonic valve.
    C. The aortic valve is to the right and lateral to the pulmonic valve.
    D. The aortic valve is to the left and anterior to the pulmonic valve.
    E. The aortic valve is to the left and posterior to the pulmonic valve.

Questions 32–35 refer to the following image of a fetus in vertex presentation with a structurally normal heart {S, D, S} and with normally related great vessels.

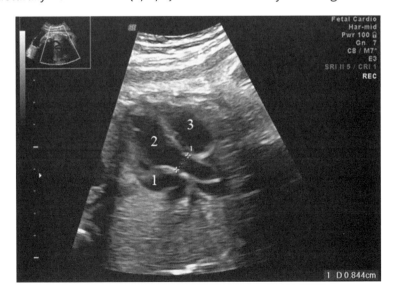

32. What structure is being measured?
    A. Tricuspid valve
    B. Pulmonic valve
    C. Ascending aorta
    D. Mitral valve
    E. Aortic valve

AIT—Hotspot item.

33. Number 1 represents the:
    A. Left atrium
    B. Right atrium
    C. Left ventricle
    D. Right ventricle
    E. Pulmonary vein

AIT—Hotspot item.

34. Number 2 represents the:
    A. Left atrium
    B. Right atrium
    C. Left ventricle
    D. Right ventricle
    E. Moderator band

AIT—Hotspot item.

35. Number 3 represents the:
    A. Left atrium
    B. Right atrium
    C. Left ventricle
    D. Right ventricle
    E. Moderator band

AIT—Hotspot item.

36. Which structures drain into the right atrium in a normal fetal heart?
    A. Superior and inferior venae cavae
    B. Coronary sinus
    C. Pulmonary veins
    D. A and B
    E. All of the above

37. What heart structure is normally seen in the left atrioventricular groove?
    A. Coronary sinus
    B. Persistent left superior vena cava
    C. Azygos vein
    D. Pulmonary vein
    E. Left ventricular outflow tract

38. What heart view is best for evaluation of the fetal coronary sinus?
    A. Short-axis view of the great arteries
    B. Short-axis view of the ventricles
    C. Apical four-chamber view
    D. Five-chamber view
    E. Aortic arch view

39. Which vessel supplies blood flow to the left ventricle and left atrium?
    A. Left coronary artery
    B. Right coronary artery
    C. Left superior vena cava
    D. Subclavian artery
    E. Ascending aorta

40. Which artery originates from the left side of the ascending aorta at the level of the aortic root and has two major branches that supply blood flow to the heart muscle?
    A. Ductus arteriosus
    B. Ductus venosus
    C. Abdominal aorta
    D. Azygos artery
    E. Left coronary artery

Questions 41–43 refer to the following image of a fetus with all heart structures normally located. The fetus is in vertex presentation.

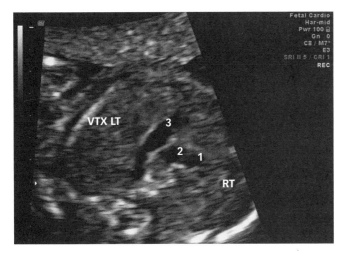

41. Number 1 represents the:
    A. Aorta
    B. Superior vena cava
    C. Main pulmonary artery
    D. Ductus arteriosus
    E. Inferior vena cava

AIT—Hotspot item.

42. Number 2 represents the:
    A. Aorta
    B. Superior vena cava
    C. Main pulmonary artery
    D. Ductus arteriosus
    E. Inferior vena cava

AIT—Hotspot item.

43. Number 3 represents the:
    A. Aorta
    B. Superior vena cava
    C. Ductus arteriosus
    D. Main pulmonary artery
    E. Inferior vena cava

AIT—Hotspot item.

44. What structures form the ductal arch?
    A. The pulmonary artery, ascending aorta, and pulmonic valve
    B. The ductus arteriosus, ascending aorta, and innominate artery
    C. The pulmonary artery, ductus arteriosus, and descending aorta
    D. The pulmonary artery, ductus arteriosus, and ascending aorta
    E. The ductus arteriosus, ascending aorta, and descending aorta

45. What vessel in the fetal circulation takes the majority of right ventricular blood flow from the pulmonary artery, allowing most of the blood to bypass the fetal lungs?
    A. Aorta
    B. Superior vena cava
    C. Left pulmonary artery
    D. Ductus arteriosus
    E. Ductus venosus

46. During a segmental exam for fetal position and situs, what is the hypoechoic organ positioned in the left upper abdomen below the fetal diaphragm in the normal fetus?
    A. Gallbladder
    B. Spleen
    C. Liver
    D. Stomach
    E. Hepatic vein

47. When determining fetal situs, you should evaluate the spleen as well as the liver. Where is the spleen located in a normal fetus?
    A. Left retroperitoneal cavity
    B. Left pelvic cavity
    C. Left upper abdomen below the diaphragm
    D. Right upper abdomen below the diaphragm
    E. Right pelvic cavity

48. To rule out isomerism, what must you note when scanning through the fetal abdomen during a fetal echocardiography exam?
    A. Spleen
    B. Liver
    C. Aorta
    D. Inferior vena cava
    E. All the above

49. When the trachea is displaced, the differential diagnosis should include a right-sided aortic arch. What sonographic view should be obtained to make this diagnosis?
    A. Apical four-chamber view
    B. Subcostal four-chamber view
    C. Long-axis view of the aorta
    D. Three-vessel view
    E. Short-axis view of the great arteries

50. The normal fetal heart occupies the following percentage of the thoracic cavity area:
    A. 15%
    B. 25%
    C. ≤33%
    D. 50%
    E. ≥75%

51. The fetal trachea and esophagus should be evaluated during a scan through the fetal thorax. What are the sonographic features of the esophagus?
    A. The esophagus appears as a tubular echogenic structure with a pattern of two echogenic lines.
    B. The esophagus bifurcates at the main bronchus.
    C. The size of the esophagus varies with fetal swallowing.
    D. A and C.
    E. All the above.

52. The initial step in any fetal echocardiographic exam is to:
    A. Establish fetal position
    B. Establish the sex of the fetus
    C. Identify the fetal stomach location
    D. Identify the arch sidedness
    E. Identify the ventricles

53. After identifying the fetal position and right and left orientation, the next step in the sequential segmental analysis is to:
    A. Identify the aortic arch sidedness
    B. Identify the location and orientation of the heart apex
    C. Identify the location of the esophagus
    D. Identify the sex of the baby
    E. All of the above

54. Which term describes a fetal heart that is situated in the fetal right chest with the apex pointing to the left?
    A. Dextrocardia
    B. Mesocardia
    C. Dextroposition
    D. Levocardia
    E. Levorotation

55. All of the following are normal levopositions EXCEPT:
    A. 20 degrees
    B. 45 degrees
    C. 25 degrees
    D. 65 degrees
    E. 35 degrees

56. Which of these terms describes the apex of the heart pointing to the fetal left chest with the axis at 45 degrees?
    A. Mesocardia
    B. Levocardia
    C. Dextrocardia
    D. Levorotation
    E. Dextroposition

57. In this image the fetus is in a vertex presentation. The heart position indicates:

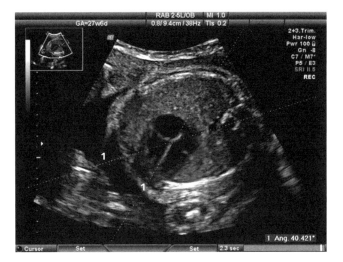

    A. Dextrocardia
    B. Dextroposition
    C. Mesocardia
    D. Levocardia
    E. Levorotation

58. What is the most leftward structure in the fetal heart?
    A. Aorta
    B. Mitral valve

    C. Tricuspid valve

    D. Main pulmonary artery

    E. Superior vena cava

59. When you are scanning through the normal fetal heart in the subcostal four-chamber heart view, what structure or structures should you see entering the left atrium?

    A. Pulmonary veins

    B. Superior vena cava

    C. Inferior vena cava

    D. Aortic arch

    E. Coronary sinus

60. Which of the following is TRUE with regard to the normal pulmonary artery and its valve?

    A. The pulmonary artery bifurcates into right and left pulmonary branches.

    B. The pulmonic valve lies anterior to the aortic valve.

    C. The pulmonary artery crosses over the aorta anteriorly.

    D. The pulmonary artery is larger than the aorta.

    E. All of the statements above are true.

61. In a normal fetal heart how many pulmonary veins normally drain into the left atrium?

    A. 1

    B. 2

    C. 3

    D. 4

    E. 5

62. The normal left pulmonary artery:

    A. Courses superior to the left bronchus

    B. Courses inferior to the left bronchus

    C. Is located more inferiorly than the right pulmonary artery

    D. Goes underneath the aorta

    E. All of the above

Questions 63–66 refer to the following image of a patient with a left aortic arch. The image was obtained with the fetal spine down and the fetus in vertex presentation.

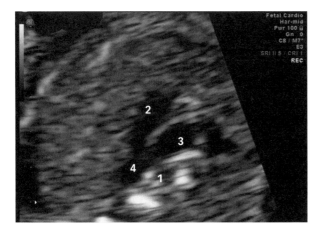

63. Number 1 represents the:
    A. Aorta
    B. Pulmonary artery
    C. Ductus arteriosus
    D. Trachea
    E. Superior vena cava

AIT—Hotspot item.

64. Number 2 represents the:
    A. Aorta
    B. Pulmonary artery
    C. Ductus arteriosus
    D. Trachea
    E. Superior vena cava

AIT—Hotspot item.

65. Number 3 represents the:
    A. Aorta
    B. Pulmonary artery
    C. Ductus arteriosus
    D. Trachea
    E. Superior vena cava

AIT—Hotspot item.

66. Number 4 represents the:
    A. Right pulmonary artery
    B. Left pulmonary artery
    C. Trachea
    D. Ductus arteriosus
    E. Superior vena cava

AIT—Hotspot item.

Questions 67–70 refer to the following image of a normal fetal heart.

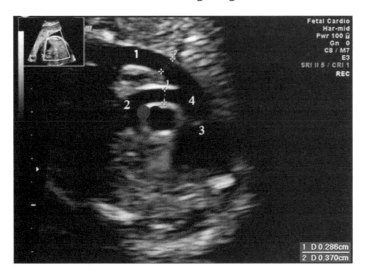

67. Number 1 represents the:
    A. Left atrium
    B. Right atrium
    C. Right pulmonary artery
    D. Patent ductus arteriosus
    E. Main pulmonary artery

AIT—Hotspot item.

68. Number 2 represents the:
    A. Left atrium
    B. Right atrium
    C. Right pulmonary artery
    D. Left pulmonary artery
    E. Main pulmonary artery

AIT—Hotspot item.

69. Number 3 represents the:
    A. Pulmonic valve
    B. Left atrium
    C. Right atrium
    D. Right pulmonary artery
    E. Left pulmonary artery

AIT—Hotspot item.

70. Number 4 represents the:
    A. Left atrium
    B. Right atrium
    C. Right pulmonary artery
    D. Main pulmonary artery
    E. Left pulmonary artery

AIT—Hotspot item.

71. When evaluating the fetal abdomen in a transverse plane at the level of the stomach, the examiner sees what vessel to the right of the aorta, just anterior to the fetal spine, in the normal fetus?
    A. Hepatic vein
    B. Superior vena cava
    C. Inferior vena cava
    D. Celiac artery
    E. Superior mesenteric artery

72. Which vessel allows blood to bypass the liver in the fetal circulation?
    A. Ductus venosus
    B. Portal vein
    C. Ductus arteriosus
    D. Umbilical vein
    E. Umbilical artery

73. Multiple echoes within the right atrium can represent the:
    A. Foramen ovale flap
    B. Eustachian valve
    C. Chiari network
    D. Tricuspid valve leaflets
    E. Both B and C

74. Which of the following functions as the pacemaker of the heart?
    A. Bundle of His
    B. Purkinje fibers
    C. Atrioventricular node
    D. Sinoatrial node
    E. Coronary sinus

75. The E/A wave ratio of the mitral valve:
    A. Remains constant throughout the pregnancy
    B. Decreases with advancing pregnancy
    C. Increases with advancing pregnancy
    D. Fluctuates with advancing pregnancy
    E. None of the above

76. The normal range for the E/A ratio is:
    A. 0.5–1.0
    B. 1.1–1.5
    C. 1.5–2.0
    D. 2.0–3.0
    E. Constant at 1.5

77. What is a normal fetal heart rate in the second trimester?
    A. Less than 60 beats per minute
    B. 60–80 beats per minute
    C. 80–100 beats per minute
    D. 100–180 beats per minute
    E. Greater than 180 beats per minute

78. Which statement about fetal heart rate is NOT true?
    A. Fetal heart rate begins between 22 and 23 days' gestation.
    B. Fetal heart rate remains constant throughout gestation.
    C. Fetal heart rate can be detected using M-mode sonography.
    D. After week 15 fetal heart rate normally ranges between 100 and 180 beats per minute.
    E. Fetal heart rate varies depending on fetal activity and rest.

79. Fetal gas exchange takes place:
    A. In the umbilical vein
    B. In the umbilical artery
    C. Through the ductus arteriosus

D. In the fetal lungs

E. In the placenta

80. Normal fetal circulation:

A. Is in series

B. Decreases with gestational age

C. Is in parallel

D. Is the same as a neonatal circulation

E. None of the above

81. The normal patent ductus arteriosus in utero:

A. Shunts blood right to left

B. Shunts blood from the pulmonary artery to the aorta

C. May be constricted with indomethacin

D. Has a normal pulsatility index of 1.9–3.0

E. All of the above

82. Which vessel in the fetal circulation regulates the amount of blood flow to the heart and liver, therefore preventing overload of volume to the fetal heart?

A. Ductus venosus

B. Ductus arteriosus

C. Inferior vena cava

D. Portal vein

E. Hepatic vein

83. The majority of blood flow entering the right atrium shunts to the left atrium via the:

A. Coronary sinus

B. Sinus venosus

C. Pulmonary veins

D. Patent foramen ovale

E. Pulmonary artery

84. What enzyme is released by the neonatal lungs shortly after birth, stimulating the closure of the ductus arteriosus?

A. Prostaglandin E

B. Bradykinin

C. Digoxin

D. Potassium

E. Carbon dioxide

85. The ductus venosus is the fetal shunt that directs blood from the umbilical vein to the fetal heart. What vessel connects the ductus venosus to the heart?

A. Superior vena cava

B. Inferior vena cava

C. Pulmonary artery

D. Pulmonary vein

E. Ductus arteriosus

86. Which of the following statements is TRUE regarding fetal cardiac output?
    A. Cardiac output increases with gestational age.
    B. The right ventricle ejects the majority of the cardiac output.
    C. Oxygen saturation in the umbilical vein is 80%–90%.
    D. Only A and B are correct.
    E. All of the above are correct.

87. The majority of fetal cardiac output is ejected by the:
    A. Left atrium
    B. Ductus arteriosus
    C. Right ventricle
    D. Aorta
    E. None of the above

88. Normally, the oxygen saturation of blood flowing into the fetus through the umbilical vein is:
    A. 55%
    B. 65%
    C. 75%
    D. 85%
    E. 95%

89. What is the placental oxygen saturation after the blood has circulated through the fetus and back to the placenta via the umbilical arteries?
    A. 58%
    B. 85%
    C. 45%
    D. 100%
    E. 65%

90. The blood circulation from the lungs enters the normal left atrium via the:
    A. Superior vena cava
    B. Ductus venosus
    C. Pulmonary arteries
    D. Foramen ovale
    E. Pulmonary veins

91. During embryologic development, the fourth left aortic arch and common dorsal aorta become the:
    A. Pulmonary arteries
    B. Ductal arch
    C. Definitive aorta
    D. Azygos vein
    E. Inferior vena cava

92. Abnormal looping of the heart tube to the left will result in:
    A. Hypoplastic left heart syndrome
    B. Corrected transposition of the great arteries

    C. Tetralogy of Fallot

    D. Situs inversus totalis

    E. Both A and C

93. During what window in fetal heart development does the fetal heart begin to beat?

    A. 7–10 days

    B. 12–14 days

    C. 21–28 days

    D. 28–35 days

    E. 35–48 days

94. In the sequence of fetal heart development, what is last to form embryologically?

    A. Truncus arteriosus

    B. Semilunar valves

    C. Bulbus cordis

    D. Coronary sinus

    E. Paired heart tube

95. A fully septated fetal heart is achieved by gestational week:

    A. 4

    B. 6

    C. 8

    D. 10

    E. 12

96. Four separate pulmonary veins are formed when the left and right pulmonary veins are absorbed. The four pulmonary veins then normally enter into the:

    A. Coronary sinus

    B. Left ventricle

    C. Right ventricle

    D. Left atrium

    E. Right atrium

97. Endocardial cushions are involved in the development of the:

    A. Semilunar valves

    B. Atrioventricular valves

    C. Membranous septum

    D. Both A and B

    E. All of the above

98. What syndrome is thought to be a result of a midline development field defect?

    A. Polysplenia syndrome

    B. Asplenia syndrome

    C. Ivemark syndrome

    D. Right atrial isomerism

    E. All of the above

99. The period of organogenesis occurs between which weeks of gestation?
    A. 0 and 3
    B. 3 and 6
    C. 4 and 8
    D. 8 and 10
    E. 10 and 12

100. If the primitive heart tube loops to the right the result is:
    A. A normal great artery relationship (d-ventricular loop)
    B. Ventricular inversion
    C. Corrected transposition of the great arteries (l-ventricular loop)
    D. Situs inversus
    E. Bilateral right-sidedness

101. The partitioning of the embryonic fetal heart into the chambers of the atria and ventricles begins at approximately what gestational day?
    A. Unknown
    B. Day 16
    C. Day 18
    D. Day 22
    E. Day 28

102. Coarctation of the aorta is thought to be the result of:
    A. Aberrant ductal tissue
    B. Decreased blood flow through the aortic isthmus
    C. Failure of the fourth and sixth aortic arches to connect with the descending aorta
    D. A and B only
    E. All of the above

103. According to the guidelines of the American Institute of Ultrasound in Medicine, when is a fetal echocardiogram most commonly performed?
    A. At 12–16 weeks' gestation
    B. At 16–18 weeks' gestation
    C. At 18–22 weeks' gestation
    D. At 24–28 weeks' gestation
    E. After 28 weeks' gestation

104. Transvaginal fetal echocardiography may be performed as early as:
    A. 4–5 weeks' gestation
    B. 6–8 weeks' gestation
    C. 10–11 weeks' gestation
    D. 11–16 weeks' gestation
    E. The fetal heart cannot be visualized with transvaginal sonography at any gestational age.

PART 2

Pathology

Abnormal perfusion and function

Assess for signs of fetal distress in response to placental or maternal injury/insult

Evaluate for the presence of fetal cardiomyopathies

Evaluate for the presence of fetal dysrhythmias

Evaluate the aortic valve

Evaluate the mitral valve

Evaluate the pulmonary valve

Evaluate the tricuspid valve

Congenital anomalies

Evaluate for cardiac malpositioning

Evaluate for congenital cardiac septal defects

Evaluate for conotruncal abnormalities

Evaluate for left-sided cardiac anomalies

Evaluate for pulmonary venous anomalies

Evaluate for right-sided cardiac anomalies

Evaluate for systemic venous anomalies

Evaluate for the presence of congenital cardiac masses

Evaluate the fetus for sonographic signs related to various genetic syndromes

105. Which dysrhythmia is most likely brought on by maternal stress or fever?
    A. Sinus tachycardia
    B. Atrial flutter
    C. Supraventricular tachycardia
    D. Ventricular tachycardia
    E. Premature atrial contraction

106. What is the definition of *fetal hydrops*?
    A. Pericardial effusion only
    B. Fluid seen in two or more fetal body cavities
    C. Fluid seen in one fetal body cavity
    D. Pleural effusion only
    E. Fluid seen in at least three fetal body cavities

107. Cardiomyopathies account for approximately what percentage of all cases of heart disease in live-born patients?
    A. Less than 1%
    B. 2%
    C. 10%
    D. 20%
    E. 30%

108. In order to assess heart function in cases of cardiomyopathy, systolic heart function must be evaluated. What is considered a normal left ventricular systolic shortening fraction (SF)?
    A. 0.10
    B. 0.15
    C. 0.20
    D. 0.25
    E. 0.30

109. What form of cardiomyopathy is associated with endocardial fibroelastosis?
    A. Dilated
    B. Hypertrophic
    C. Restrictive
    D. Both A and D
    E. All of the above

110. Hypertrophic cardiomyopathies are generally associated with all of the following EXCEPT:
    A. Fetal anemias
    B. Maternal diabetes
    C. Noonan syndrome
    D. Glycogen storage disease
    E. Twin-to-twin transfusion syndrome

111. The most common type of cardiomyopathy is:
    A. Hypertrophic
    B. Restrictive
    C. Congestive
    D. Dilated
    E. C and D

112. What maternal disease is most commonly associated with hypertrophic cardiomyopathy?
    A. Maternal diabetes
    B. Maternal lupus erythematosus
    C. Glycogen storage disorder
    D. CMV (cytomegalovirus)
    E. Rubella

113. This image demonstrates:

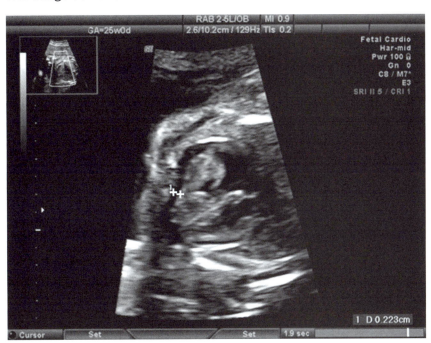

    A. Congestive cardiomyopathy
    B. Dilated cardiomyopathy
    C. Hypertrophic cardiomyopathy
    D. Restrictive cardiomyopathy
    E. Both A and B

AIT—Hotspot item.

See 402
Pericardial
effusion

114. All of the following views may be helpful in evaluating fetal arrhythmias EXCEPT the:
    A. Long-axis view of the aorta
    B. Short-axis view of the great vessels
    C. Short-axis view of the ventricles
    D. Apical five-chamber view
    E. Apical four-chamber view

115. Which syndrome is associated with a complex heart defect in 95%–100% of cases, may progress to bradycardia and complete heart block, and has a high mortality rate?
    A. Noonan syndrome
    B. Patau syndrome (trisomy 13)
    C. Ivemark syndrome
    D. Asplenia syndrome
    E. Polysplenia syndrome

116. Ebstein anomaly is commonly associated with which fetal dysrhythmia?
    A. Premature atrial contractions
    B. Supraventricular tachycardia
    C. Bradycardia
    D. Sinus tachycardia
    E. Atrial bigeminy

117. Cardiomyopathies can be associated with what dysrhythmia?
    A. Bradycardia
    B. Complete heart block
    C. Supraventricular tachycardia
    D. A and B only
    E. A, B, and C

118. Which dysrhythmia is characterized by a nonconducted premature atrial contraction that occurs every other beat?
    A. Sinus bradycardia
    B. Atrial bigeminy
    C. Ventricular tachycardia
    D. Premature atrial contraction
    E. Premature ventricular contraction

119. A heart rhythm with an early atrial beat that is NOT followed by a ventricular beat is considered:
    A. Blocked premature atrial contraction
    B. Complete atrioventricular block
    C. Partial atrioventricular block
    D. Premature atrial contraction
    E. Supraventricular tachycardia

120. Which of the following is considered the most common fetal dysrhythmia?
    A. Bradycardia
    B. Premature atrial contractions
    C. Premature ventricular contractions
    D. Supraventricular tachycardia
    E. Complete heart block

121. An atrial heart rate of 300–500 beats per minute with varying ventricular response suggests:
    A. Atrial bigeminy
    B. Atrial flutter
    C. Ventricular tachycardia
    D. Sinus tachycardia
    E. Premature atrial contractions

122. A fetus has a heart rate of 198 beats per minute with normal atrioventricular activation. This presentation suggests:
    A. Normal fetal heart rate
    B. Supraventricular tachycardia
    C. Sinus tachycardia
    D. Ventricular tachycardia
    E. Premature ventricular contraction

123. Which of these dysrhythmias has an early atrial beat that is NOT followed by a ventricular beat?
    A. Complete heart block
    B. Partial atrioventricular block
    C. Sinus bradycardia
    D. Nonconducted premature atrial contraction
    E. Nonconducted premature ventricular contraction

124. The most common type of pathologic tachycardia is:
    A. Sinus tachycardia
    B. Ventricular tachycardia
    C. Atrial flutter
    D. Supraventricular tachycardia
    E. Premature atrial contraction

125. What describes dissociation between atrial and ventricular complexes, with the atrial rate being faster than the ventricular rate?
    A. Atrial bigeminy
    B. Complete heart block
    C. Sinus bradycardia
    D. Premature atrial contractions
    E. Supraventricular tachycardia

126. With pathologic bradycardia, 96% of the patients have:
    A. Second-degree heart block
    B. Third-degree heart block (complete heart block)
    C. Atrial bigeminy
    D. Sinus bradycardia
    E. Both A and B

127. Which of the following defines atrial fibrillation?
   A. Atrial rate greater than ventricular rate
   B. Atrial rate of 300–500 beats per minute
   C. Regular ventricular rate
   D. Variable ventricular rate
   E. All of the above

128. All of the following lesions have abnormal blood flow and are considered progressive heart lesions EXCEPT:
   A. Aortic stenosis
   B. Pulmonic stenosis
   C. Hypoplastic left heart syndrome
   D. L-transposition of the great arteries
   E. Coarctation of the aorta

129. The most common type of aortic stenosis is:
   A. Valvular aortic stenosis
   B. Subvalvular aortic stenosis
   C. Supravalvular aortic stenosis
   D. Aortic atresia
   E. None of the above

130. Endocardial fibroelastosis, small left ventricle, mitral stenosis, and small aorta are all features of this heart lesion seen in the pediatric population:
   A. Atrial septal defect
   B. Ventricular septal defect
   C. Pulmonary stenosis
   D. Aortic valve stenosis
   E. Patent ductus arteriosus

131. In this image the waveform labeled 1 is acquired with the fetus in a vertex presentation. There is no visible heart defect. The pulse wave being measured represents:

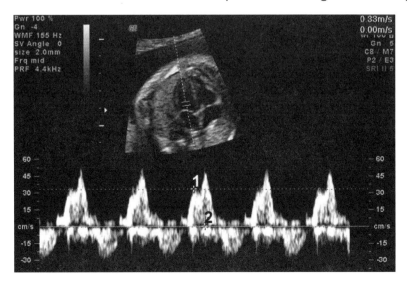

A. E-wave tricuspid valve

B. E-wave mitral valve

C. A-wave tricuspid valve

D. A-wave mitral valve

E. Left ventricular outflow tract

AIT—Hotspot item.

132. If the diameter of the pulmonary orifice is 50%–80% of the aortic orifice diameter, what abnormality exists?
   A. Mild to moderate aortic stenosis.
   B. Mild to moderate aortic insufficiency.
   C. Mild to moderate pulmonary stenosis.
   D. Severe pulmonary stenosis.
   E. None of the above; this is within normal limits.

133. What fetal heart view is ideal to evaluate for pulmonic valve insufficiency?
   A. Apical long-axis view of the pulmonary artery
   B. Apical four-chamber view
   C. Subcostal four-chamber view
   D. Short-axis view of the great vessels
   E. A and D

134. Embryologic pulmonic stenosis occurs because of:
   A. Cell death abnormality
   B. Tissue-migration abnormality
   C. Extracellular matrix abnormality
   D. Abnormal intracardiac blood flow
   E. Abnormal targeted growth

135. What is the most common type of pulmonic stenosis?
   A. Valvular pulmonic stenosis
   B. Subvalvular pulmonic stenosis
   C. Branch pulmonary artery stenosis
   D. Supravalvular pulmonic stenosis
   E. A and B equally

136. The heart defect most commonly associated with double-outlet right ventricle is:
   A. Atrial septal defect
   B. Right ventricular hypertrophy
   C. Aortic stenosis
   D. Pulmonic stenosis
   E. Right-sided aortic arch

137. The definition of *tricuspid atresia* is:
   A. Dysplastic tricuspid valve
   B. Partial agenesis of the tricuspid valve

    C. Complete agenesis of the tricuspid valve

    D. Hypoplasia of the tricuspid valve

    E. Apically displaced tricuspid valve

138. Tricuspid atresia is commonly associated with:

    A. Ventricular septal defects

    B. Pulmonary atresia/stenosis

    C. Hypoplasia of the right ventricle

    D. A, B, and C

    E. B and C

139. The most common morphologic variant of the tricuspid valve associated with tricuspid atresia is:

    A. Muscular atresia of the right atrial floor

    B. Membranous atresia

    C. Valvular atresia

    D. Ebstein anomaly

    E. Common atrioventricular canal

140. Tricuspid atresia is classified into three types based on:

    A. Presence of an atrial septal defect

    B. The relationship of the great arteries

    C. Degree of narrowing of the tricuspid valve

    D. Presence of flow across the tricuspid valve

    E. Degree of hypoplasia of the right ventricle

141. With tricuspid atresia where is the pulmonary artery in relation to the aorta?

    A. Superior and to the right

    B. Anterior and to the right

    C. Anterior and to the left

    D. Posterior and to the left

    E. Posterior and to the right

142. All of the following will cause an enlarged right atrium, but which condition is the only one that includes an apically displaced tricuspid valve?

    A. Tricuspid insufficiency

    B. Ebstein anomaly

    C. Uhl anomaly

    D. Tricuspid atresia

    E. Tricuspid stenosis

143. What is the most common great artery relationship in tricuspid valve atresia?

    A. Type I, normally related great arteries

    B. Type II, d-transposition

    C. Type III, l-transposition

    D. Type IV, equally distributed

    E. Type V, side-by-side great arteries

144. A massively enlarged right atrium is identified with an apically displaced tricuspid valve. This most likely represents what cardiac heart defect?
    A. Uhl malformation
    B. Tricuspid atresia
    C. Ebstein anomaly
    D. Hypoplastic right heart syndrome
    E. Hypoplastic left heart syndrome

145. In Ebstein anomaly, which leaflet has a sail-like appearance?
    A. Anterior leaflet of tricuspid valve
    B. Posterior leaflet of tricuspid valve
    C. Septal leaflet of mitral valve
    D. Both A and B
    E. All of the above

146. The risk of a heart defect in cases of situs inversus with extreme levocardia is:
    A. 2%
    B. 10%
    C. 25%
    D. 90%
    E. Nearly 100%

147. If the fetal abdominal organs are properly arranged but the fetal heart is positioned in the right chest, the risk that the fetus has a heart defect is:
    A. 2%
    B. 10%
    C. 25%
    D. 95%
    E. 100%

148. What is the risk for a heart defect if the fetal situs is situs solitus?
    A. Less than 1%
    B. 2%
    C. 75%
    D. 95%
    E. Nearly 100%

149. When the fetal heart is in the right thorax and the abdominal organs are NOT properly arranged, the fetal situs would be:
    A. Situs solitus
    B. Situs inversus
    C. Visceral situs inversus
    D. Situs ambiguus
    E. Visceral situs solitus

150. Ectopia cordis is a heart defect that may be associated with which of the following malformations?
    A. Pentalogy of Cantrell
    B. Limb–body wall complex
    C. Amniotic band syndrome
    D. A and B
    E. A, B, and C

151. All of the following are associated with extreme levocardia EXCEPT:
    A. Hypoplastic left heart syndrome
    B. Tetralogy of Fallot
    C. Ebstein anomaly
    D. Truncus arteriosus
    E. Double-outlet right ventricle

152. Situs ambiguus is also known as:
    A. Levoposition
    B. Levorotation
    C. Dextrocardia
    D. Dextroposition
    E. Heterotaxy

153. An abnormal heart position in the fetal chest may be caused by:
    A. Congenital pulmonary airway malformation
    B. Congenital diaphragmatic hernia
    C. Bronchopulmonary sequestration
    D. Pleural effusion
    E. All of the above

154. What is the most common congenital heart defect other than a bicuspid aortic valve?
    A. Atrial septal defect
    B. Ventricular septal defect
    C. Aortic stenosis
    D. Atrioventricular septal defect
    E. Pulmonic stenosis

155. Atrial septal defects constitute what percentage of all congenital heart defects?
    A. 2.0%
    B. 5.4%
    C. 6.7%
    D. 8.0%
    E. Greater than 10%

156. Of all newborns with a congenital heart defect, what percentage have aortic stenosis?
    A. 1%–2%
    B. 3%–6%

C. 8%–10%

D. 12%–15%

E. 20%–25%

157. An ostium secundum atrial septal defect is caused by:
   A. Excessive reabsorption of the septum primum
   B. Excessive reabsorption of the septum secundum
   C. Incomplete fusion of the endocardial cushions
   D. Both B and C
   E. Both A and C

158. By definition, which of the following cardiac lesions has a hemodynamic communication between the right and left ventricles?
   A. Septum primum atrial septal defect
   B. Ventricular septal defect
   C. Patent foramen ovale
   D. Semilunar valve
   E. Septum secundum atrial septal defect

159. What is the most commonly recognized cardiac defect?
   A. Ventricular septal defect
   B. Atrial septal defect
   C. Atrioventricular septal defect
   D. Bicuspid aortic valve
   E. Pulmonic stenosis

160. In tetralogy of Fallot, the most common location of the ventricular septal defect is:
   A. Subaortic
   B. Apical
   C. Subpulmonic
   D. Both A and B
   E. None of the above

161. The most common type of atrial septal defect is:
   A. Sinus venosus
   B. Ostium secundum
   C. Ostium primum
   D. Coronary sinus
   E. Trabecular defect

162. What type of atrial septal defect generally occurs as part of a more complex type of congenital heart defect such as an atrioventricular canal defect?
   A. Ostium secundum
   B. Sinus venosus
   C. Ostium primum
   D. Coronary sinus
   E. Trabecular defect

163. Which anomaly accounts for approximately 30%–50% of all fetal congenital heart defects?
    A. Ventricular septal defect
    B. Hypoplastic left heart syndrome
    C. Atrial septal defect
    D. Coarctation of the aorta
    E. Aortic stenosis

164. What type of interrupted aortic arch is commonly associated with a ventricular septal defect?
    A. Type A
    B. Type B
    C. Type C
    D. Type D
    E. Type E

165. What cardiac lesion is most common in a fetus with double-outlet right ventricle?
    A. Ventricular septal defect
    B. Aortic stenosis
    C. Atrial septal defect
    D. Pulmonary stenosis
    E. Partial anomalous pulmonary venous return

166. The most common location for a ventricular septal defect in a fetus with double-outlet right ventricle is:
    A. Subaortic
    B. Doubly committed
    C. Subpulmonary
    D. Remote
    E. Both A and C

167. The most common type of ventricular septal defect is:
    A. Inlet
    B. Trabecular
    C. Muscular
    D. Outlet
    E. Membranous

168. The most common location for a ventricular septal defect in double-outlet left ventricle is:
    A. Subaortic
    B. Subpulmonic
    C. Doubly committed
    D. Remote
    E. Noncommitted

169. What congenital heart defect is associated with subvalvular aortic stenosis?
    A. Ventricular septal defect
    B. Coarctation of the aorta
    C. Interrupted aortic arch
    D. Both B and C
    E. All of the above

170. This image demonstrates: *(See Color Plate 1 on page xvii.)*

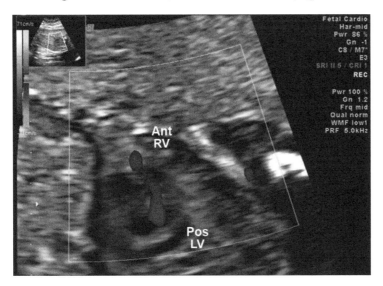

    A. Atrial septal defect
    B. Membranous ventricular septal defect
    C. Muscular ventricular septal defect
    D. Coronary sinus
    E. Atrioventricular septal defect
AIT—Hotspot item.

171. Which cardiac heart defect is demonstrated in this image?

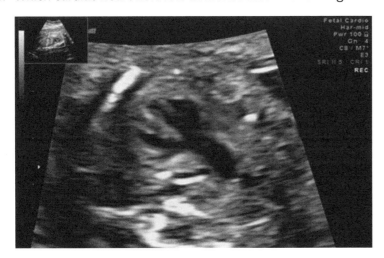

    A. Tetralogy of Fallot with pulmonary atresia
    B. Truncus arteriosus

    C. Double-outlet right ventricle with pulmonary atresia

    D. Differential diagnoses would include all of the above

    E. None of the above

172. A persistent left superior vena cava is often associated with:
    A. Ostium primum atrial septal defect
    B. Sinus venosus atrial septal defect
    C. Ostium secundum atrial septal defect
    D. Coronary sinus atrial septal defect
    E. Atrioventricular septal defect

173. Univentricular heart accounts for the following percentage of all cardiac heart defects:
    A. Less than 1%
    B. 1%–3%
    C. 4%–6%
    D. 8%–10%
    E. 12%–20%

174. All of the following are considered tissue-migration abnormalities EXCEPT:
    A. Double-outlet right ventricle
    B. Tetralogy of Fallot
    C. Pulmonic stenosis
    D. Truncus arteriosus
    E. D-transposition of the great arteries

175. Which of the following defects is NOT thought to result from cell death abnormalities?
    A. Ostium primum atrial septal defect
    B. Muscular ventricular septal defect
    C. Ebstein anomaly
    D. Atrioventricular septal defect
    E. Both A and D

176. Embryologically, an atrioventricular septal defect is considered a/an:
    A. Extracellular matrix abnormality
    B. Abnormal intracardiac blood flow abnormality
    C. Tissue-migration abnormality
    D. Cellular death abnormality
    E. Targeted growth abnormality

177. This congenital heart defect results from the failure of the endocardial cushions to fuse properly:
    A. Atrial septal defect
    B. Univentricular heart
    C. Ventricular septal defect
    D. Atrioventricular septal defect
    E. Hypoplastic left heart syndrome

178. The most common embryologic tissue-migration abnormality is:
     A. Double-outlet right ventricle
     B. Tetralogy of Fallot
     C. Pulmonic stenosis with ventricular septal defect
     D. D-transposition of the great arteries
     E. Truncus arteriosus

179. What heart lesion is in most cases due to disturbances in bulboventricular loop
     development during the embryonic stage?
     A. Asplenia
     B. Polysplenia
     C. Univentricular heart
     D. Atrioventricular septal defect
     E. Ventricular septal defect

180. Which of the following heart defects is considered to be a conotruncal heart defect?
     A. Diaphragmatic hernia
     B. Atrioventricular septal defect
     C. Ebstein anomaly
     D. Coarctation of the aorta
     E. Tetralogy of Fallot

181. All of the following are considered to be conotruncal heart defects EXCEPT:
     A. Pulmonary atresia with an intact interventricular septum
     B. Double-outlet right ventricle
     C. Truncus arteriosus
     D. Transposition of the great arteries
     E. Ventricular septal defect

182. What cardiac heart lesion is associated with abnormal looping of the heart tube?
     A. Ebstein anomaly
     B. Atrioventricular septal defect
     C. Polysplenia
     D. Tetralogy of Fallot
     E. Ventricular septal defect

183. What cardiac defect is classified by the pulmonary artery or arteries originating off a
     single great vessel arising from the heart?
     A. Truncus arteriosus
     B. Hypoplastic left heart syndrome
     C. Double-outlet right ventricle
     D. Patent ductus arteriosus
     E. Pulmonic atresia

184. In truncus arteriosus, a single truncal valve *may* arise, but is *least likely* to arise, over the:
    A. Ventricular septal defect
    B. Left ventricle
    C. Right ventricle
    D. Aorta
    E. Pulmonary artery

185. What is the most common type of atrioventricular septal defect in the live-born?
    A. Complete
    B. Indeterminate/transitional
    C. Incomplete/partial
    D. Mixed
    E. Both A and C

186. In d-transposition of the great arteries, the aorta:
    A. Is connected to the left ventricle
    B. Overrides a ventricular septal defect
    C. Is connected to the right ventricle
    D. Is connected to the pulmonary artery
    E. Is connected to the left atrium

187. In l-transposition of the great arteries:
    A. The aorta is connected to the morphologic right ventricle
    B. The morphologic right ventricle is the most anterior structure
    C. The ventricles are inverted
    D. Both A and C
    E. A, B, and C

188. Univentricular heart is classified by the presence or absence of:
    A. A moderator band
    B. Atrioventricular valves
    C. A rudimentary ventricular chamber
    D. Both B and C
    E. All of the above

189. In truncus arteriosus the truncal valve most commonly consists of the following number of cusps:
    A. 2 cusps
    B. 3 cusps
    C. 4 cusps
    D. 5 cusps
    E. 0 cusps

190. The Collett and Edwards classification of truncus arteriosus is based on:
    A. The origin of the aorta
    B. The relationship of the great arteries
    C. The number of truncal cusps

D. The origin of the pulmonary arteries

E. Presence of truncal insufficiency

191. In both corrected and complete transposition of the great arteries, what is connected to the morphologic right ventricle?
    A. Pulmonary artery
    B. Aorta
    C. Tricuspid valve
    D. Mitral valve
    E. Bicuspid valve

192. In both corrected and complete transposition of the great arteries, what is connected to the morphologic left ventricle?
    A. Aorta
    B. Mitral valve
    C. Tricuspid valve
    D. Pulmonary artery
    E. Bicuspid valve

193. With transposition of the great arteries, which of these fetal heart views will be abnormal?
    A. Apical four-chamber view
    B. Subcostal four-chamber view
    C. Short-axis view of the great vessels
    D. Long-axis view of the great vessels
    E. Both C and D

194. What is the most common abnormality in children born with cyanotic heart disease?
    A. Truncus arteriosus
    B. Double-outlet right ventricle
    C. D-transposition of the great arteries
    D. Tetralogy of Fallot
    E. Univentricular heart

195. With d-transposition of the great arteries, postnatal circulation is best described as:
    A. Normal
    B. Series
    C. Reverse
    D. Parallel
    E. Restrictive

196. With l-transposition of the great arteries, postnatal circulation is best described as:
    A. Normal
    B. Series
    C. Reverse
    D. Parallel
    E. Restrictive

197. What cardiac heart defect is demonstrated in this image?

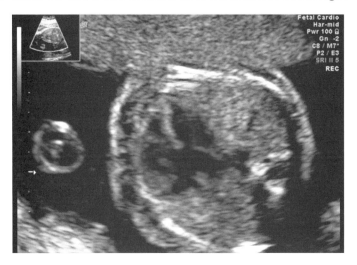

    A. Ebstein anomaly

    B. Ventricular septal defect

    C. Atrial septal defect

    D. Atrioventricular septal defect

    E. Hypoplastic left heart syndrome

AIT—Hotspot item.

198. This fetus in breech presentation demonstrates:

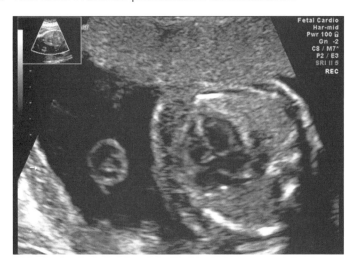

    A. Ventricular inversion

    B. Ventricular disproportion

    C. Atrioventricular valves at the same level

    D. Hypoplastic right heart

    E. Hypoplastic left heart syndrome

199. The great vessels will be seen parallel to each other in all of the following cardiac heart defects EXCEPT:

    A. Double-outlet right ventricle

    B. Tetralogy of Fallot

    C. D-transposition of the great arteries

    D. L-transposition of the great arteries

    E. Double-outlet left ventricle

200. With abnormal intracardiac blood flow and volume through the left side of the heart, all of the following lesions could be seen EXCEPT:

    A. Hypoplastic left heart syndrome

    B. Aortic valve stenosis

    C. Mitral valve atresia

    D. Pulmonary atresia

    E. Coarctation of the aorta

201. Hypoplastic left heart syndrome is associated with all of the following conditions EXCEPT:

    A. Aortic atresia

    B. Hypoplastic aorta

    C. Double-outlet right ventricle

    D. Small left ventricle

    E. Coarctation of the aorta

202. Which form of interrupted aortic arch is the most common?

    A. Type A

    B. Type B

    C. Type C

    D. Type I

    E. Type II

203. In double-outlet right ventricle associated with tetralogy of Fallot, the great vessel relationship is:

    A. Normally related great arteries

    B. Side-by-side great arteries

    C. Dextromalposed aorta

    D. Levomalposed aorta

    E. Juxtomalposed great arteries

204. The cardiac anomaly most commonly associated with hypoplastic left heart syndrome is:

    A. Coarctation of the aorta

    B. Endocardial fibroelastosis

    C. Interrupted aortic arch

    D. Pulmonic stenosis

    E. Tachycardia

205. In coarctation of the aorta, the aortic narrowing occurs at what level approximately 98% of the time?

    A. Between the innominate artery and the left common carotid artery

    B. Distal to the ductal arch

    C. Between the left common carotid artery and the subclavian artery

    D. Between the left subclavian artery and the ductus arteriosus

    E. Between the ascending aorta and the innominate artery

206. Of the four classic features of tetralogy of Fallot, which is generally NOT seen in utero?
   A. Ventricular septal defect
   B. Overriding aorta
   C. Pulmonic stenosis
   D. Right ventricular hypertrophy
   E. All of the above are commonly seen in utero.

207. What is the most common cardiac cause of death in the early neonate?
   A. Atrial septal defect
   B. Complete heart block
   C. Hypoplastic right heart syndrome
   D. Hypoplastic left heart syndrome
   E. Patent ductus arteriosus

208. Coarctation of the aorta is found in 70% of patients with:
   A. Tricuspid atresia
   B. Hypoplastic left heart syndrome
   C. Mitral stenosis
   D. Both B and C
   E. All of the above

209. What is the most common associated cardiac defect in a fetus with coarctation of the aorta?
   A. Aortic stenosis
   B. Mitral stenosis
   C. Mitral atresia
   D. Bicuspid aortic valve
   E. Pulmonic stenosis

210. A fetus with aortic atresia is seen with a poorly contracting left ventricle. The walls appear hyperechoic and the left ventricle is dilated. This presentation describes:
   A. Complete heart block
   B. Turner syndrome
   C. Endocardial fibroelastosis
   D. Ebstein anomaly
   E. Both B and C

211. All of the following are classic features of tetralogy of Fallot EXCEPT:
   A. Aortic stenosis
   B. Overriding aorta
   C. Perimembranous ventricular septal defect
   D. Pulmonic stenosis
   E. Right ventricular hypertrophy

212. What is the most severe form of obstructive lesion of the left side of the heart?
   A. Aortic atresia
   B. Mitral atresia
   C. Hypoplastic left heart syndrome
   D. Coarctation of the aorta
   E. All of the above

213. Which of the following is considered a ventricular inflow abnormality?
   A. Cor triatriatum
   B. Parachute mitral valve
   C. Supravalvular mitral ring
   D. A, B, and C
   E. None of the above

214. What is a common indirect sign of coarctation of the aorta?
   A. Left ventricular hyperplasia
   B. Right ventricular diameter greater than left ventricular diameter
   C. Left ventricular diameter greater than right ventricular diameter
   D. Bicuspid aortic valve
   E. Heart shift to the right

215. What cardiac heart defect is seen in this image?

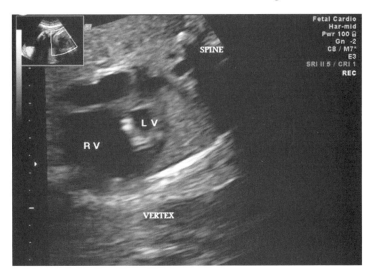

   A. Endocardial fibroelastosis
   B. Hypoplastic left heart
   C. Hypoplastic right heart
   D. Both A and B
   E. Both A and C

AIT—Hotspot item.

216. Univentricular heart is divided into four groups, the most common of which is:
    A. Complex univentricular heart with asplenia
    B. Complex univentricular heart with polysplenia
    C. Double-inlet single ventricle, left ventricle morphology
    D. Double-inlet single ventricle, right ventricle morphology
    E. Complete univentricle, single-inlet, right ventricle morphology

217. What cardiac anomaly is demonstrated by two of the great arteries coming off the left ventricle?
    A. Double-outlet right ventricle
    B. Double-outlet left ventricle
    C. Corrected transposition of the great arteries
    D. Truncus arteriosus
    E. Complete transposition of the great arteries

218. This image demonstrates:

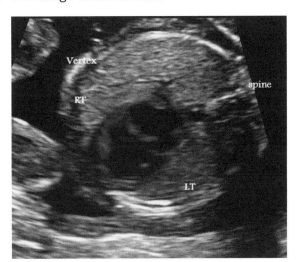

    A. Univentricular heart
    B. Tetralogy of Fallot
    C. Ebstein anomaly
    D. Pericardial effusion
    E. Normal heart
AIT—Hotspot item.

219. Which type of univentricular heart is most lethal?
    A. Type A
    B. Type B
    C. Type C
    D. Type D
    E. Type E

220. This drawing represents which type of aortic arch abnormality?

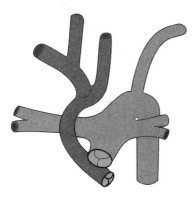

    A. Type A interruption
    B. Type B interruption
    C. Type C interruption
    D. Preductal coarctation
    E. Postductal coarctation

221. What is the least frequent occurrence of interrupted aortic arch?
    A. Type A interruption
    B. Type B interruption
    C. Type C interruption
    D. Preductal coarctation
    E. Postductal coarctation

222. With severe hypoplastic left heart syndrome, you would expect to see all of the following in the intracardiac fetal heart survey EXCEPT:
    A. Small left ventricle
    B. Enlarged right heart
    C. Right-to-left shunting at the atrial level
    D. Left-to-right shunting at the atrial level
    E. Hypoplastic aorta

223. In total anomalous pulmonary venous return (TAPVR) there will always be:
    A. An atrial septal defect
    B. A ventricular septal defect
    C. A right-to-left shunt at the atrial level
    D. Both A and C
    E. A, B, and C

224. What is the most common type of total anomalous pulmonary venous return (TAPVR)?
    A. Supracardiac
    B. Infracardiac
    C. Cardiac
    D. Mixed
    E. Partial

225. Infracardiac partial anomalous pulmonary venous connection is associated with:
    A. Shone syndrome
    B. Scimitar syndrome
    C. Cor triatriatum
    D. Situs inversus
    E. Heterotaxy syndrome

226. Partial anomalous pulmonary venous connection from the right lung is almost always present with:
    A. Ostium primum atrial septal defect
    B. Sinus venosus atrial septal defect
    C. Ostium secundum atrial septal defect
    D. Coronary sinus atrial septal defect
    E. Atrioventricular septal defect

227. One of the first signs of total anomalous pulmonary venous return (TAPVR) in the fetus is:
    A. Enlarged right ventricle
    B. Prominent pulmonary artery
    C. Enlarged left ventricle
    D. Both A and B
    E. All of the above

228. Which type of total anomalous pulmonary venous return (TAPVR) is almost always associated with a severe obstruction?
    A. Supracardiac
    B. Cardiac
    C. Infracardiac
    D. Mixed anomalous
    E. Partial anomalous

229. This type of total anomalous pulmonary venous return (TAPVR) is rarely obstructed:
    A. Supracardiac
    B. Cardiac
    C. Infracardiac
    D. Mixed anomalous
    E. Partial anomalous

230. The cardiac defect found in all cases of total anomalous pulmonary venous return (TAPVR) is:
    A. Atrial septal defect
    B. Ventricular septal defect
    C. Left superior vena cava
    D. Right-sided aortic arch
    E. Coarctation of the aorta

231. What type of atrial septal defect is almost always present with partial anomalous pulmonary venous return?
    A. Ostium secundum atrial septal defect
    B. Ostium primum atrial septal defect
    C. Sinus venosus atrial septal defect
    D. Coronary sinus atrial septal defect
    E. None of the above

232. An enlarged right atrium and apically displaced tricuspid valve are classic features of what congenital heart defect?
    A. Ebstein anomaly
    B. Hypoplastic left heart syndrome
    C. Double-outlet right ventricle
    D. Pulmonic stenosis
    E. Tetralogy of Fallot

233. Classic features of this heart defect include a plate-like pulmonic valve, massive distention of the pulmonary artery and its branches, and commonly a right-sided aortic arch:
    A. Pulmonary stenosis
    B. Absent pulmonic valve syndrome
    C. Agenesis of the ductus venosus
    D. Tetralogy of Fallot
    E. Truncus arteriosus

234. Hypoplasia of the right ventricle most commonly results from:
    A. Tricuspid stenosis
    B. Ventricular septal defect
    C. Redundant foramen ovale
    D. Pulmonary atresia with an intact interventricular septum
    E. Mitral valve insufficiency

235. What cardiac defect is most commonly associated with double-outlet right ventricle (DORV)?
    A. Pulmonary stenosis
    B. Aortic stenosis
    C. Tricuspid stenosis
    D. Mitral stenosis
    E. Total anomalous pulmonary venous return

236. If the ventricular septum bows toward the left ventricle, what does this indicate?
    A. Severe tricuspid regurgitation
    B. Severe mitral regurgitation
    C. Ebstein anomaly
    D. A and C
    E. All of the above

237. The cardiac defect most commonly associated with truncus arteriosus is:
    A. Right-sided aortic arch
    B. Agenesis of the ductus arteriosus
    C. Pulmonary stenosis
    D. Atrial septal defect
    E. Persistent left superior vena cava

238. The most common relationship of the great vessels in double-outlet right ventricle is:
    A. Normal
    B. Dextromalposed
    C. Side by side
    D. Levomalposed
    E. Single great vessel

239. Which of the following has been associated with a right-sided aortic arch?
    A. Pulmonary atresia
    B. Truncus arteriosus
    C. Tetralogy of Fallot
    D. D-transposition of the great arteries
    E. All of the above

240. If there is a complex heart defect and the aorta is seen overriding the left ventricle by more than 50%, the defect may be:
    A. Pulmonary atresia with ventricular septal defect
    B. Tetralogy of Fallot
    C. Truncus arteriosus
    D. Double-outlet right ventricle
    E. All of the above

241. The most common type of double-outlet right ventricle is:
    A. Double-outlet right ventricle with a subaortic ventricular septal defect
    B. Double-outlet right ventricle with a subpulmonic ventricular septal defect
    C. Double-outlet right ventricle with a doubly committed ventricular septal defect
    D. Double-outlet right ventricle with a remote ventricular septal defect
    E. Double-outlet right ventricle with no ventricular septal defect

242. Classic Taussig-Bing heart is a combination of:
    A. Subpulmonic atrial septal defect with side-by-side great vessels
    B. Subpulmonic ventricular septal defect with side-by-side great vessels
    C. Remote ventricular septal defect with normal great vessels
    D. Subaortic ventricular septal defect with normal great vessels
    E. Subaortic ventricular septal defect with side-by-side great vessels

243. More than 65%–70% of cases of double-outlet right ventricle are associated with the following cardiac anomaly:
    A. Aortic stenosis
    B. Left ventricular hypoplasia
    C. Atrial septal defect
    D. Pulmonic stenosis
    E. Coarctation of the aorta

244. This image demonstrates what cardiac heart defect?

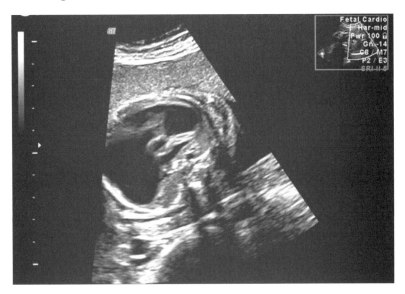

    A. Ebstein anomaly (dysplastic tricuspid valve)
    B. Univentricular heart
    C. Atrioventricular septal defect
    D. Total anomalous venous return
    E. Pericardial effusion

AIT—Hotspot item.

245. In more than 60% of cases the condition illustrated in question 244 is associated with:
    A. Ventricular septal defect
    B. Transposition of the great arteries
    C. Atrial septal defect
    D. Aortic stenosis or atresia
    E. Pulmonic stenosis

246. Exposure to which of the following drugs is thought to be associated with the cardiac heart defect in question 244?
    A. Cocaine
    B. Indomethacin
    C. Lithium
    D. Amphetamines
    E. Alcohol

247. The differential diagnosis for the anomaly demonstrated in the two images below would include all of the following EXCEPT: *(See Color Plate 2 on page xvii.)*

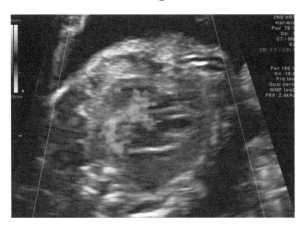 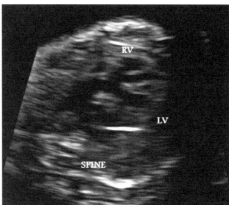

A. Secundum atrial septal defect

B. Ventricular septal defect

C. Overriding aorta

D. Truncus arteriosus

E. Tetralogy of Fallot

248. The cardiac heart defect illustrated in question 247 would be considered a/an:

A. Abnormal intracardiac blood flow abnormality

B. Extracellular matrix abnormality

C. Abnormal targeted growth abnormality

D. Tissue-migration abnormality

E. Cell death abnormality

249. What cardiac heart defect is demonstrated in this drawing?

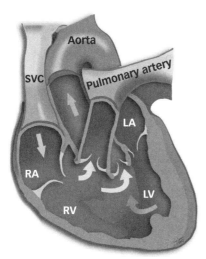

A. Double-outlet right ventricle

B. Tetralogy of Fallot

C. Trabecular ventricular septal defect

D. Atrioventricular septal defect

E. Double-outlet left ventricle

250. This image demonstrates:

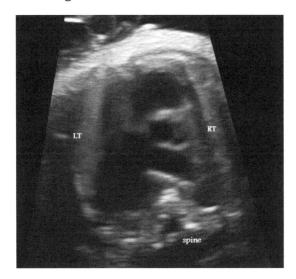

   A. Dilated aorta
   B. Dilated pulmonary arteries
   C. Dilated inferior vena cava
   D. Normal three-vessel view
   E. Bicuspid aortic valve

AIT—Hotspot item.

251. The image in question 250 demonstrates a classic feature of:
   A. Aortic stenosis
   B. Pulmonic stenosis
   C. Absent pulmonic valve syndrome
   D. Double-outlet right ventricle
   E. Truncus arteriosus

252. You see two vessels posterior to the heart in the four-chamber heart view. What anomaly do you suspect?
   A. Tetralogy of Fallot
   B. Interrupted inferior vena cava with azygos vein continuation
   C. Truncus arteriosus
   D. Right atrial isomerism
   E. Tricuspid atresia

253. Which of the following syndromes is associated with an interrupted inferior vena cava and an azygos vein continuation?
   A. Asplenia
   B. Double-outlet right ventricle
   C. Univentricular heart
   D. Polysplenia
   E. Turner syndrome

(and atrial Septal Defects)

254. With a sinus venosus defect of the superior vena cava, 80%–90% of fetuses will have what defect?
    A. Ventricular septal defect
    B. Bicuspid aortic valve
    C. Anomalous pulmonary venous connections
    D. Interrupted inferior vena cava
    E. Agenesis of the ductus venosus

255. When a dilated inferior vena cava is seen, the suspected diagnosis would be:
    A. Single umbilical artery
    B. Bicuspid aortic valve
    C. Anomalous pulmonary venous connections
    D. Interrupted inferior vena cava
    E. Agenesis of the ductus venosus

256. Where would a coronary sinus atrial septal defect be located?
    A. Atrial septum
    B. Left ventricle
    C. Right ventricle
    D. Left atrium
    E. Right atrium

257. A coronary sinus atrial septal defect is generally associated with:
    A. Left superior vena cava
    B. Tetralogy of Fallot
    C. Ventricular septal defect
    D. Total anomalous pulmonary venous connection
    E. Partial anomalous pulmonary venous connection

258. What is the most common cardiac venous anomaly?
    A. Azygos vein continuation
    B. Absent ductus venosus
    C. Interrupted inferior vena cava
    D. Umbilical vein aneurysm
    E. Persistent left superior vena cava

259. In a four-chamber heart view, a round cyst-like structure in the left atrium may indicate:
    A. Left atrial aneurysm
    B. Persistent left superior vena cava
    C. Dilated pulmonary vein
    D. Rhabdomyoma
    E. Redundant foramen ovale

260. A dilated coronary sinus may be associated with:
    A. Interrupted inferior vena cava
    B. Absent ductus venosus

C. Persistent left superior vena cava

D. Azygos vein

E. Umbilical vein aneurysm

261. In this image what cardiac heart structure is being marked with the calipers?

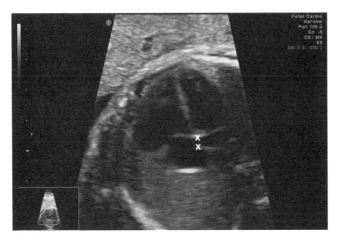

A. Foramen ovale

B. Right atrium

C. Secundum atrial septal defect

D. Dilated coronary sinus

E. Eustachian valve

AIT—Hotspot item.

262. In this image the arrow points to the following structure:

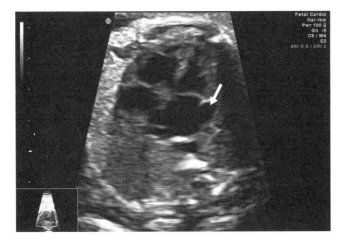

A. Right atrium

B. Persistent left superior vena cava

C. Left atrial cyst

D. Eustachian valve

E. Redundant foramen ovale

AIT—Hotspot item.

263. In this image, the fetus is in a vertex presentation with spine toward the maternal right. What does this image demonstrate?

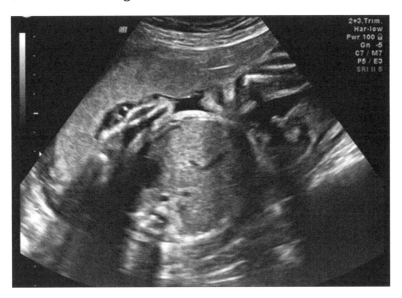

A. Normal umbilical vein
B. Persistent left umbilical vein
C. Persistent right umbilical vein
D. Normal ductus venosus
E. Agenesis of the ductus venosus

264. Which syndrome is associated with an interrupted inferior vena cava and an azygos vein continuation?
A. Asplenia syndrome
B. Ivemark syndrome
C. Left atrial isomerism
D. Polysplenia syndrome
E. Both C and D

265. The most common cardiac tumor found in a fetus is:
A. Rhabdomyoma
B. Teratoma
C. Hemangioma
D. Fibroma
E. Myxoma

266. Rhabdomyomas are commonly associated with:
A. Echogenic foci
B. Pulmonic stenosis
C. Myxoma
D. Maternal diabetes
E. Tuberous sclerosis

267. What heart lesion is defined by a large lobulated cystic mass attached to the base of the heart by a stalk and accompanied by pericardial effusion?
    A. Rhabdomyoma
    B. Fibroma
    C. Intrapericardial teratoma
    D. Hemangioma
    E. Myxoma

268. Which of the following cardiac tumors is generally NOT found in a fetus?
    A. Rhabdomyoma
    B. Hemangioma
    C. Myxoma
    D. Fibroma
    E. Teratoma

269. Which of the following is NOT considered a cardiac tumor?
    A. Echogenic foci
    B. Hemangioma
    C. Myxoma
    D. Fibroma
    E. Rhabdomyoma

270. What is another name for polysplenia syndrome?
    A. Bilateral right-sidedness
    B. Left atrial isomerism
    C. Bilateral left-sidedness
    D. Shone syndrome
    E. Both B and C

271. Atrial septal defects are commonly associated with the following syndrome:
    A. Turner syndrome
    B. Holt-Oram syndrome (heart-hand syndrome)
    C. Williams syndrome
    D. Noonan syndrome
    E. Patau syndrome (trisomy 13)

272. Which of the following syndromes describes a fetus with abnormal situs, multiple spleens, and both atria with left atrial features?
    A. Asplenia syndrome
    B. Polysplenia syndrome
    C. Ivemark syndrome
    D. Edwards syndrome
    E. Shone syndrome

273. Which congenital heart defect has a strong association with aneuploidy?
    A. Atrioventricular septal defect
    B. Tetralogy of Fallot
    C. Double-outlet right ventricle
    D. All of the above
    E. A and B only

274. Turner syndrome is associated with:
    A. Coarctation of the aorta
    B. Aortic stenosis
    C. Hypoplastic left heart syndrome
    D. A and B
    E. All of the above

275. What syndrome is commonly associated with a dysplastic pulmonic valve?
    A. Turner syndrome
    B. Trisomy 18 (Edwards syndrome)
    C. Noonan syndrome
    D. DiGeorge syndrome
    E. Trisomy 13 (Patau syndrome)

276. Complete heart block with an atrioventricular septal defect is suggestive of:
    A. Asplenia syndrome
    B. Polysplenia syndrome
    C. Ivemark syndrome
    D. Down syndrome
    E. Patau syndrome

277. Atrioventricular septal defect with tetralogy of Fallot is associated with:
    A. Down syndrome (trisomy 21)
    B. Patau syndrome (trisomy 13)
    C. Edwards syndrome (trisomy 18)
    D. Polysplenia syndrome
    E. Asplenia syndrome

278. Atrioventricular septal defect with double-outlet right ventricle is associated with:
    A. Down syndrome (trisomy 21)
    B. Edwards syndrome (trisomy 18)
    C. Patau syndrome (trisomy 13)
    D. Polysplenia syndrome
    E. Asplenia syndrome

279. The inferior vena cava is seen anterior to the aorta in the four-chamber view. This is suggestive of:
    A. Asplenia syndrome
    B. Left atrial isomerism

C. Polysplenia syndrome

D. Right atrial isomerism

E. A and D

280. What syndrome would most commonly be associated with this image?

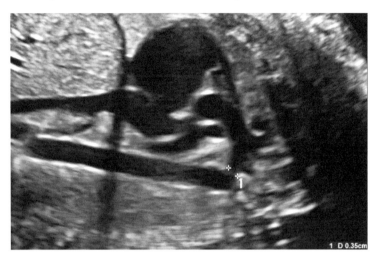

A. Noonan syndrome

B. Down syndrome (trisomy 21)

C. Turner syndrome

D. Asplenia syndrome

E. Polysplenia syndrome

281. The syndrome most commonly associated with the cardiac heart defect shown here is:

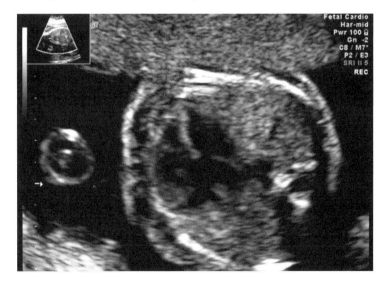

A. Down syndrome (trisomy 21)

B. Asplenia syndrome

C. Polysplenia syndrome

D. Ivemark syndrome

E. All of the above

282. Univentricular heart is often associated with:
    A. Edwards syndrome (trisomy 18)
    B. Asplenia syndrome
    C. Polysplenia syndrome
    D. Coarctation of the aorta
    E. All of the above

283. If a Type B aortic arch abnormality is combined with a ventricular septal defect, 50% or more of these cases will be associated with what syndrome?
    A. Williams syndrome
    B. Noonan syndrome
    C. Down syndrome
    D. DiGeorge syndrome
    E. Asplenia syndrome

284. Supravalvular aortic stenosis is associated with:
    A. Turner syndrome
    B. Edwards syndrome (trisomy 18)
    C. Williams syndrome
    D. Down syndrome (trisomy 21)
    E. Patau syndrome (trisomy 13)

285. Pulmonic stenosis is associated with:
    A. Edwards syndrome (trisomy 18)
    B. Noonan syndrome
    C. Down syndrome (trisomy 21)
    D. Both A and B
    E. All of the above

286. Which of the following syndromes is associated with truncus arteriosus?
    A. Williams syndrome
    B. Noonan syndrome
    C. Turner syndrome
    D. DiGeorge syndrome
    E. Down syndrome (trisomy 21)

287. What syndrome is associated with an atrioventricular septal defect and double-outlet right ventricle?
    A. Polysplenia syndrome
    B. Asplenia syndrome
    C. DiGeorge syndrome
    D. Left atrial isomerism
    E. Shone syndrome

288. All of the following are associated with Shone syndrome EXCEPT:
    A. Parachute mitral valve
    B. Subaortic stenosis
    C. Supravalvular mitral membrane
    D. Cor triatriatum
    E. Coarctation of the aorta

289. Another name for asplenia syndrome is:
    A. Bilateral right-sidedness
    B. Right atrial isomerism
    C. Ivemark syndrome
    D. Both A and B
    E. All of the above

290. Complete heart block with an atrioventricular septal defect is associated with:
    A. Asplenia syndrome
    B. Trisomy 21 (Down syndrome)
    C. Polysplenia syndrome
    D. Both B and C
    E. All of the above

291. What syndrome is associated with double-outlet right ventricle, atrioventricular canal defect, total anomalous pulmonary venous return, and right-sided heart obstruction?
    A. Left atrial isomerism
    B. Right atrial isomerism
    C. Ebstein anomaly
    D. Edwards syndrome (trisomy 18)
    E. Shone syndrome

292. What syndrome is associated with an interrupted inferior vena cava and left-sided heart obstruction?
    A. Polysplenia syndrome
    B. Asplenia syndrome
    C. Edwards syndrome
    D. Ivemark syndrome
    E. Shone syndrome

293. Noonan syndrome is commonly associated with what cardiac lesion?
    A. Mitral atresia
    B. Coarctation of the aorta
    C. Pulmonic valve stenosis
    D. Aortic stenosis
    E. Aortic atresia

294. When increased nuchal translucency persists into the second trimester, this thickening is termed a *nuchal cystic hygroma*. Of fetuses with cystic hygroma persisting into the second trimester, 75% have a chromosomal abnormality. In this group, what is the most common abnormality?
    A. Patau syndrome
    B. Edwards syndrome
    C. Klinefelter syndrome
    D. Turner syndrome
    E. Marfan syndrome

PART 3

Patient Care

Infection control

Maintain infection control

Practice Standard/Universal Precautions

295. The Standard (Universal) Precautions are:
    A. Actions taken to create a barrier between you and potentially infected body fluids
    B. Measures taken to prevent the transmission of blood-borne diseases
    C. Approaches to infection control
    D. Methods of preventing transmission of blood-borne diseases
    E. All of the above

296. The ultrasound technologist is required to practice proper hand hygiene. This procedure involves:
    A. Washing hands thoroughly with soap and water for 40–60 seconds after every examination.
    B. Rubbing hands completely with an alcohol-based product for 20–30 seconds until dry after every examination.
    C. Hand washing only if gloves are not worn during the examination.
    D. Hand washing or rubbing only if the technologist contacts body fluids or secretions during the ultrasound examination.
    E. Either A or B is acceptable.

297. If a patient presents for a fetal echocardiographic examination and has a raised rash on her abdomen, what should you as the sonographer do?
    A. Postpone the examination until the rash resolves.
    B. Avoid scanning over the infected area.
    C. Perform the examination wearing protective gloves.
    D. Clean the transducer after the procedure with a recommended equipment disinfectant.
    E. Both C and D.

298. What precautions should you take during an endovaginal exam to reduce the transmission of infectious diseases?
    A. Wear gloves.
    B. Cover the transducer with an approved commercial probe cover.
    C. Clean and sanitize the probe.
    D. All of the above.
    E. Only A and B.

299. Which of the following is potentially infectious?
    A. Blood
    B. Vaginal fluid
    C. Synovial fluid
    D. Cerebrospinal fluid
    E. All of the above

300. Which of the following is NOT among the Standard Precautions to which you should adhere for a fetal echocardiographic examination?
   A. Wearing gloves during every examination
   B. Cleaning and disinfecting the ultrasound transducer after every examination
   C. Wearing protective clothing and eyewear
   D. Discarding used linens in an approved linen bag after every examination
   E. Maintaining proper hand hygiene

301. In the United States, what agency is responsible for overseeing all healthcare facilities and ensuring that their employees follow the practices stipulated by the Standard Precautions?
   A. Federal Emergency Management Agency (FEMA)
   B. Occupational Safety and Health Administration (OSHA)
   C. American Registry for Diagnostic Medical Sonography (ARDMS)
   D. American Hospital Association (AHA)
   E. Centers for Disease Control (CDC)

PART 4

Integration of Data

Incorporate outside data

Assess indications for performing a fetal echocardiogram

Obtain pertinent medical history of patient

Use chromosomal anomalies or genetic syndromes as exam indicators

Use family history as exam indicator

Use fetal clinical signs and symptoms to guide the echocardiogram

Use fetal dysrhythmias as exam indicators

Use fetal extracardiac malformations as exam indicators

Use hydrops as exam indicator

Use maternal diseases as exam indicators

Use maternal drug exposure as exam indicators

Use suspected cardiac abnormality on an outside scan as exam indicator

Use thickened nuchal translucency as exam indicator

Reporting results

Compare echocardiographic results to other imaging modalities

302. All of the following are indications for a fetal echocardiographic exam EXCEPT:
    A. Family history of congenital heart defect
    B. History of tuberous sclerosis
    C. Extracardiac abnormality
    D. Echogenic foci
    E. Exposure to teratogenic medications

303. Of all live-born infants, how many will have a cardiac defect?
    A. 1 in 1000 infants
    B. 4 in 1000 infants
    C. 6 in 1000 infants
    D. 8 in 1000 infants
    E. 10 in 1000 infants

304. As an isolated heart defect, which of the following is the most commonly recognized cardiac lesion, accounting for about 30% of all cardiac defects recognized in live-borns?
    A. Atrial septal defect
    B. Coarctation of the aorta
    C. Ventricular septal defect
    D. Atrioventricular septal defect
    E. Aortic stenosis

305. Maternal diabetes is an indication for performing a fetal echocardiogram. Type II diabetes mellitus is defined as an increased Hgb A1C level of at least:
    A. 2.5%
    B. 4.0%
    C. 6.5%
    D. 8.0%
    E. 10.0%

306. When there are multiple tumors in the right and left ventricles of the fetal heart and the patient has a history of tuberous sclerosis, what cardiac tumor should be suspected?
    A. Teratoma
    B. Myxoma
    C. Fibroma
    D. Rhabdomyoma
    E. Hemangioma

307. Of all infants born with a congenital heart defect, what percentage of these infants will have an abnormal karyotype?
    A. 1%–5%
    B. 8%
    C. 13%
    D. 35%
    E. 50%

308. What percentage of patients with trisomy 21 (Down syndrome) have congenital heart defects?
    A. 10%
    B. 25%
    C. 50%
    D. 75%
    E. 100%

309. What chromosomal abnormality is associated with an atrioventricular septal defect in at least 40% of the cases?
    A. Trisomy 21 (Down syndrome)
    B. Trisomy 13 (Patau syndrome)
    C. Trisomy 18 (Edwards syndrome)
    D. Turner syndrome
    E. Noonan syndrome

310. In which of these syndromes will there be a congenital heart defect almost 100% of the time?
    A. Turner syndrome
    B. Trisomy 13 (Patau syndrome)
    C. Trisomy 21 (Down syndrome)
    D. Trisomy 18 (Edwards syndrome)
    E. Both B and D

311. When truncus arteriosus is diagnosed, which syndrome is associated in 21% of the cases?
    A. DiGeorge syndrome
    B. Down syndrome (trisomy 21)
    C. Turner syndrome
    D. Noonan syndrome
    E. Edwards syndrome (trisomy 18)

312. If there were a family history of a syndrome, which would warrant a fetal echocardiographic exam?
    A. Marfan syndrome
    B. DiGeorge syndrome
    C. Holt-Oram syndrome (heart-hand syndrome)
    D. A and B only
    E. All of the above

313. What is the recurrence risk for a congenital heart defect if two or more siblings are affected?
    A. No increased risk
    B. 2%–4%
    C. 10%
    D. 15%–20%
    E. >20%

314. What is the recurrence risk for a congenital heart defect when the mother of the baby is affected?
    A. No increased risk
    B. 2%–4%
    C. 10%–12%
    D. 15%–20%
    E. >20%

315. What is the recurrence risk for a congenital heart defect when a single sibling is affected?
    A. No increased risk
    B. 2%–4%
    C. 10%–12%
    D. 15%–20%
    E. >20%

316. What cardiac heart defect has the highest recurrence rate?
    A. Ventricular septal defect
    B. Atrial septal defect
    C. Bicuspid aortic valve
    D. Univentricular heart
    E. Transposition of the great arteries

317. Of the fetal findings listed below, which one would NOT be an indication for a fetal heart examination?
    A. Oligohydramnios
    B. Polyhydramnios
    C. Bradycardia
    D. Intrauterine growth restriction
    E. A fetal heart rate of 230 beats per minute

318. Why is nonimmune fetal hydrops an indication for fetal echocardiography?
    A. It suggests the presence of structural heart defects.
    B. It suggests complications from Rh isoimmunization.
    C. It indicates the presence of alloimmune hemolytic disease.
    D. It may indicate fetal cardiac dysrhythmias.
    E. A and D.

319. The risk for congenital heart disease is increased in a fetus with a nuchal translucency thickness that exceeds:
    A. 1.5 mm
    B. 2.5 mm
    C. 3.5 mm
    D. 4.5 mm
    E. 5.5 mm

320. A healthy pregnant female presents for a routine obstetric ultrasound exam, and the fetal heart rate is 350 beats per minute with a varying ventricular rate. These findings suggest:
    A. Sinus tachycardia
    B. Supraventricular tachycardia
    C. Atrial flutter
    D. Ventricular tachycardia
    E. Blocked premature atrial contraction

321. Noncardiac fetal anomalies detected on a routine exam may indicate an increased risk for a complex heart defect in that fetus. Which fetal anomaly, if found in isolation, would NOT warrant further evaluation with a fetal echocardiography exam?
    A. Omphalocele
    B. Gastroschisis
    C. Renal agenesis
    D. Dandy-Walker malformation
    E. Diaphragmatic hernia

322. Polysplenia is associated with other cardiac anomalies in the following percentage of cases:
    A. 8%–10%
    B. 10%–12%
    C. 25%–45%
    D. 50%–60%
    E. 90%–95%

323. In what percentage of cases is duodenal atresia associated with a congenital heart defect?
    A. 5.2%
    B. 17.1%
    C. 25.4%
    D. 52.0%
    E. 78.0%

324. During a routine fetal exam, the fetus is diagnosed with multiple limb–body wall abnormalities, including an omphalocele, hydrocephalus, and scoliosis. What would be the most common heart defect associated with this condition?
    A. Rhabdomyoma
    B. Univentricular heart
    C. Ectopia cordis
    D. Truncus arteriosus
    E. Ventricular septal defect

325. What is the most common cause of nonimmune hydrops fetalis?
    A. Cardiomyopathy-induced arrhythmias
    B. Ebstein anomaly
    C. Asplenia syndrome
    D. Polysplenia syndrome
    E. Atrioventricular septal defect

326. Which of the following maternal conditions is NOT an indication for a fetal echocardio-graphic exam?
    A. Maternal diabetes
    B. Maternal connective tissue disorder
    C. Maternal use of alcohol
    D. Maternal hyperthyroidism
    E. Maternal hyperphenylalaninemia (phenylketonuria)

327. A patient has a history of uncontrolled diabetes. These two images most likely demonstrate:

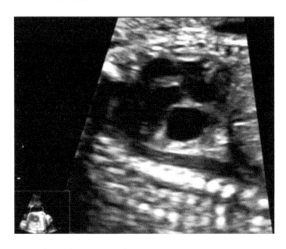 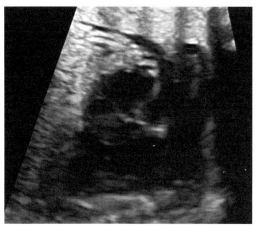

    A. Ebstein anomaly
    B. Truncus arteriosus
    C. Normal orientation of the great arteries
    D. Transposition of the great arteries
    E. Tetralogy of Fallot

328. Which maternal metabolic disorder has a high association with tetralogy of Fallot?
    A. Phenylketonuria (hyperphenylalaninemia)
    B. Type I diabetes mellitus
    C. Collagen vascular disease
    D. Hyperthyroidism
    E. Gestational diabetes

329. If you detect fetal bradycardia in utero with an atrial rate of 140 beats per minute (bpm) and a ventricular rate of 40 bpm, the mother should be tested for:
    A. Antibodies specific for SSA/Ro and SSB/La
    B. Rubella
    C. Measles
    D. HIV
    E. Syphilis

330. Maternal pregestational diabetes is associated with:
    A. Increased risk of cardiac defects
    B. Increased risk of neural tube defects
    C. Increased risk of fetal blindness
    D. Increased risk of cleft palate
    E. Both A and B

331. Maternal systemic lupus erythematosus may present with:
    A. Premature atrial contractions
    B. Complete heart block in the fetus
    C. Premature ventricular contractions
    D. Sinus tachycardia
    E. Supraventricular tachycardia

332. Which of the following maternal infections is NOT an indication for a fetal heart exam?
    A. Human immunodeficiency virus (HIV)
    B. Rubella
    C. Cytomegalovirus
    D. Parvovirus
    E. Coxsackievirus

333. What is the most common fetal cardiac finding associated with diabetic mothers?
    A. Double-outlet left ventricle
    B. Hypertrophic cardiomyopathy
    C. Double-outlet right ventricle
    D. Truncus arteriosus
    E. Both C and D

334. There is a high incidence of complete heart block without a structural heart defect in fetuses of mothers with:
    A. Connective tissue disorder
    B. Asplenia syndrome
    C. Polysplenia syndrome
    D. Left ventricular aneurysm
    E. Pericardial effusion

335. Which infectious maternal disease is most commonly associated with pulmonary stenosis?
    A. Toxoplasmosis
    B. Cytomegalovirus
    C. Rubella
    D. Parvovirus
    E. Hepatitis B

336. When subvalvular aortic stenosis is seen in utero, it is known as *idiopathic hypertrophic subaortic stenosis*. What is most commonly associated with this condition?
    A. Maternal diabetes
    B. Maternal systemic lupus erythematosus
    C. Maternal rubella
    D. Hypertrophic cardiomyopathy
    E. Both A and D

337. What maternal condition is often associated with aortic stenosis?
    A. Rubella
    B. Diabetes
    C. Lupus erythematosus
    D. Both A and B
    E. All of the above

338. Hypertrophic cardiomyopathy is commonly associated with:
    A. Noonan syndrome
    B. Diabetic mothers
    C. Maternal glycogen storage disease
    D. Twin-to-twin transfusion syndrome
    E. All of the above

339. The heart lesion most commonly seen with exposure to teratogens is:
    A. Atrial septal defect
    B. Atrioventricular septal defect
    C. Ventricular septal defect
    D. Tetralogy of Fallot
    E. Truncus arteriosus

340. If the fetus has fetal alcohol syndrome, the risk of a cardiac anomaly is:
    A. No increased risk
    B. 2%–4%
    C. 5%–10%
    D. 25%–30%
    E. 40%–50%

341. A patient is in the third trimester and has been taking ibuprofen for the past week. What is the most likely effect on the fetal heart?
    A. Ductus arteriosus constriction
    B. Decreased systolic ventricular function
    C. Aortic stenosis
    D. Hydrops
    E. Premature atrial contractions

342. Which of these statements about indomethacin therapy is TRUE?
    A. It is a pharmacologic drug used to treat preterm labor.
    B. This drug may cause constriction of the ductus arteriosus if used for a prolonged period of time.
    C. If ductal constriction occurs indomethacin therapy should be discontinued.
    D. Ductus arteriosus constriction will regress after discontinuing indomethacin.
    E. All are true statements.

343. Maternal exposure to certain medicinal drugs increases a fetus's risk for a congenital heart defect. Which of the following drugs does NOT increase the risk of a heart defect?
    A. Thalidomide
    B. Trimethadione
    C. Lithium
    D. Nifedipine
    E. Amphetamines

344. The congenital heart defect most commonly associated with lithium exposure is:
    A. Atrial septal defect
    B. Ebstein anomaly
    C. Tricuspid atresia
    D. Uhl malformation
    E. Atrioventricular septal defect

345. Premature atrial contractions may be associated with all of the following EXCEPT:
    A. Maternal use of caffeine
    B. Redundant foramen ovale flap
    C. Use of cigarettes
    D. Maternal alcohol consumption
    E. Maternal fever

346. Maternal alcohol abuse is an indication for fetal *echocardiography* because it is associated with an increased risk for:
    A. Fetal alcohol syndrome
    B. Perinatal alcohol addiction
    C. Congenital heart defects
    D. Hypotelorism
    E. Turner syndrome

347. At what gestational age is a fetus most susceptible to teratogen exposure?
    A. 0–4 weeks
    B. 4–8 weeks
    C. 12–16 weeks
    D. 20–24 weeks
    E. 30–36 weeks

348. Which of the following maternal conditions is an indication for fetal echocardiography?
    A. In vitro fertilization
    B. 22q11.2 deletion syndrome
    C. Exposure to retinoids
    D. B and C
    E. All of the above.

349. A fetus is diagnosed with a congenital heart defect during a routine ultrasound exam. The risk that this fetus has an extracardiac defect is:
    A. 5%–10%
    B. 10%–15%
    C. 15%–25%
    D. 25%–45%
    E. 50%

350. If a fetus has a congenital heart defect diagnosed by fetal ultrasound, what is the risk that the fetus will have an abnormal karyotype?
    A. 15%
    B. 35%
    C. 50%
    D. 85%
    E. 100%

351. A healthy 25-year-old pregnant female presents for a fetal echo exam for isolated echogenic foci in the left ventricle. What is the risk of a cardiac defect?
    A. No increased risk
    B. 1%–2% risk
    C. 5%–10% risk
    D. 10%–12% risk
    E. 50%–75% risk

352. A thickened nuchal translucency identified by ultrasound is an indication for screening by fetal echocardiography. What is the appropriate time frame for performing the nuchal translucency measurement?
    A. 11–14 weeks' gestation
    B. 14–18 weeks' gestation
    C. 18–23 weeks' gestation
    D. 24–26 weeks' gestation
    E. Any gestational age

353. Of fetuses with a serious congenital heart defect, what percentage will have a thickened nuchal translucency greater than 95% for gestational age?
    A. 1%–2%
    B. 10%–15%
    C. 15%–30%
    D. 40%–50%
    E. 90%–95%

354. Fetuses with a nuchal translucency that exceeds the 99th percentile for gestational age and crown–rump length are at high risk for which of these cardiac abnormalities?
    A. Hypoplastic left heart syndrome
    B. Coarctation of the aorta
    C. Aortic stenosis
    D. None of the above
    E. A, B, and C

355. In addition to 3D real-time echocardiography, which of the following imaging modalities can be used to assess left ventricular function?
    A. 4D sonography
    B. B-mode sonography
    C. Computed tomography
    D. Continuous-wave Doppler
    E. A and D

356. Which of these imaging modalities is used as an adjunct to M-mode in assessing fetal heart rate and rhythm?
    A. B-mode
    B. Spectral Doppler
    C. Computed tomography
    D. 3D sonography
    E. Magnetic resonance imaging

357. Serial ultrasound studies are recommended in cases of *fetal congenital pulmonary airway malformation* (CPAM)—also known as *congenital cystic adenomatoid malformation* (CCAM) or *cystic adenomatoid malformation of the lung* (CAML)—to assess the mass location, size, and consequences for the cardiovascular system. What other imaging modality would be helpful in assessing the mass's size, location, and effects on surrounding structures?
    A. Computed tomography
    B. Radiography
    C. Magnetic resonance imaging
    D. Nuclear medicine
    E. Positron emission tomography

358. Compared with ultrasound, what is the utility of magnetic resonance imaging in cases of a diaphragmatic hernia?
    A. MRI can better visualize the lung/liver tissue interfaces.
    B. MRI is helpful in determining heart displacement in the fetal thorax.
    C. MRI helps determine liver position in the fetus.
    D. A and C.
    E. A, B, and C.

359. A routine scan was performed on a 32-week fetus. In the four-chamber heart view, the right ventricle was slightly larger than the left ventricle. This image was taken for further evaluation. The pulsed-wave Doppler in the descending aorta shows decreased flow signals across the area of caliper 1. Caliper 1 suggests:

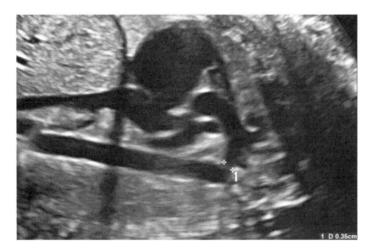

A. Normal aortic arch

B. Coarctation of the aorta

C. Dilated isthmus

D. Hypoplastic transverse aortic arch

E. Interrupted aortic arch

AIT—Hotspot item.

PART 5

Protocols

Clinical standards and guidelines

Demonstrate the cardiac five-chamber view

Demonstrate the four-chamber views

Demonstrate the long-axis views

Demonstrate the orientation of the great vessels using various cardiac views

Demonstrate the pulmonary vein and branches views

Demonstrate the short-axis views

Demonstrate the three-vessel view

Demonstrate the various views of the arches

Demonstrate the vena caval views

Use Doppler to evaluate fetal heart rate

Use M-mode to evaluate fetal heart rate

Measurement techniques

Perform fetal cardiac biometry measurements to assess visualized cardiac structures

Perform various gray-scale measurements to assess visualized cardiac structures

Perform various gray-scale measurements to assess visualized pathology

360. Which of these statements is TRUE regarding the apical five-chamber view of the normal fetal heart?
    A. The aortic and mitral valves exhibit continuity posteriorly.
    B. The aorta and interventricular septum have continuity anteriorly.
    C. The aorta arises from the center of the heart.
    D. The aorta arises between the two atrioventricular valves.
    E. All of the above are true statements.

361. Which is the best cardiac heart view for visualizing persistent truncus arteriosus?
    A. Apical four-chamber view
    B. Subcostal four-chamber view
    C. Apical five-chamber view
    D. Long-axis view of the aorta
    E. Both C and D

362. The best sonographic view for diagnosing an atrioventricular septal defect is the:
    A. Apical four-chamber view
    B. Subcostal four-chamber view
    C. Short-axis view
    D. Five-vessel view
    E. Both A and B

363. Which view best demonstrates the atrioventricular junction, including the valve leaflets and annulus?
    A. Apical four-chamber view
    B. Short-axis view
    C. Subcostal four-chamber view
    D. Five-chamber view
    E. A and C

364. The best view for evaluating a conoventricular or perimembranous ventricular septal defect is the:
    A. Apical four-chamber view
    B. Subcostal four-chamber view
    C. Long-axis view of the aorta
    D. Long-axis view of the pulmonary artery
    E. Short-axis view of the ventricles

365. What is NOT seen on the routine four-chamber view?
    A. Foramen ovale flap bulging from right atrium to left atrium
    B. Moderator band present in the right ventricle
    C. Septal attachments of the tricuspid valve to the interventricular septum
    D. Aortic wall continuity with the interventricular septum
    E. Pulmonary veins being accepted into the left atrium

366. What sonographic view was used to obtain this image?

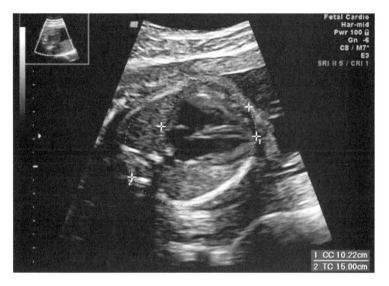

A. Short-axis view of the great vessels
B. Subcostal four-chamber view
C. Long-axis view of the aorta
D. Long-axis view of the pulmonary artery
E. Long-axis view of the great vessels

367. The four-chamber heart view has been reported to have a sensitivity of what percentage in detecting a congenital heart defect?
A. 10%–25%
B. 50%–78%
C. 85%–92%
D. 40%–57%
E. 100%

368. In the apical four-chamber heart view, how is the interventricular septum oriented in relation to the sound beam?
A. Perpendicular
B. Parallel
C. At a 90-degree angle
D. Both A and C
E. None of the above

369. Which of the following is considered a standard fetal echocardiography view?
A. Apical four-chamber view
B. Short-axis view of the great arteries
C. Long-axis view of the aorta
D. Long-axis view of the pulmonary artery
E. All of the above are considered standard views.

370. In the subcostal four-chamber view of the normal fetal heart, which cardiac structure is closest to the fetal spine?
   A. Right ventricle
   B. Left ventricle
   C. Right atrium
   D. Left atrium
   E. Mitral valve

371. What sonographic view was used to obtain this image?

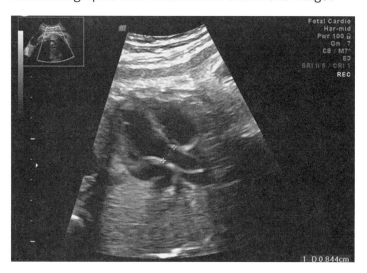

   A. Long-axis view of the aorta
   B. Long-axis view of the pulmonary artery
   C. Apical four-chamber view
   D. Subcostal four-chamber view
   E. Short-axis view of the great vessels

372. To what vessel is the arrow in this image pointing? *(See Color Plate 3 on page xviii.)*

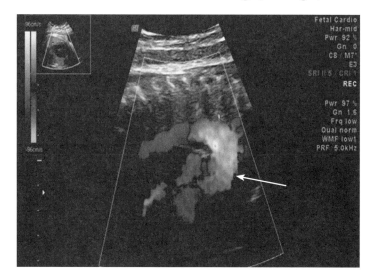

A. Pulmonary artery

B. Ductus arteriosus

C. Aortic arch

D. Inferior vena cava

E. Superior vena cava

AIT—Hotspot item.

373. In which of the following heart views can the anterior aortic wall be seen continuous with the interventricular septum in the normal fetal heart?
A. Short-axis view of the great arteries
B. Long-axis view of the aorta
C. Subcostal four-chamber view
D. Apical four-chamber view
E. Short-axis view of the ventricles

374. In the long-axis view of the left heart, which of these structures are visible?
A. Left atrium, mitral valve, and left ventricle
B. Right atrium, tricuspid valve, and papillary muscle
C. Left atrium, mitral valve, papillary muscle, right ventricle, and left ventricle
D. Left atrium, mitral valve, papillary muscle, left ventricle, and pulmonic valve
E. Papillary muscle, right ventricle, and pulmonic valve

375. List the vessels in the three-vessel view in order from the vessel with the largest diameter to the vessel with the smallest diameter in the normal thorax:
A. Pulmonary artery > superior vena cava > aorta
B. Aorta > pulmonary artery > superior vena cava
C. Superior vena cava > aorta > pulmonary artery
D. Pulmonary artery > aorta > superior vena cava
E. Aorta > superior vena cava > pulmonary artery

376. In the long-axis view of the pulmonary artery, the normal pulmonary artery courses:
A. Cephalad, leftward, and posterior to the right ventricle
B. Caudad, leftward, and posterior to the right ventricle
C. Cephalad, rightward, and anterior to the right ventricle
D. Caudad, rightward, and anterior to the right ventricle
E. Cephalad, rightward, and posterior to the right ventricle

377. The great arteries cross with the pulmonary artery and the aorta oriented at what angle to each other?
A. 135-degree angle
B. 180-degree angle
C. 90-degree angle
D. 45-degree angle
E. 25-degree angle

378. The position of the pulmonic valve in relation to the aortic valve is:
    A. Anterior and inferior
    B. Posterior and inferior
    C. Posterior and superior
    D. Anterior and superior
    E. At the same level

379. When scanning through the fetal heart, at what level do you determine the normal great artery position?
    A. Where the aorta and pulmonary artery cross
    B. At the level of the three-vessel view
    C. At the level of the semilunar valves
    D. None of the above
    E. Both A and C

380. The fetus in this image is in the vertex presentation, spine down, and had a normal fetal heart scan. The white arrows identify the: *(See Color Plate 4 on page xviii.)*

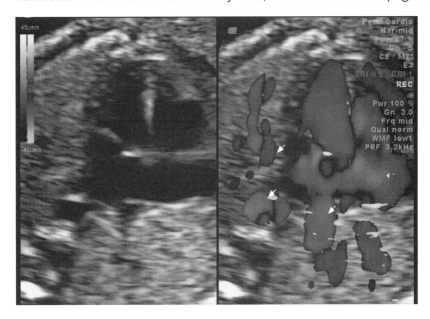

    A. Persistent left superior vena cava
    B. Right superior vena cava
    C. Pulmonary artery
    D. Prominent inferior vena cava
    E. Pulmonary veins

AIT—Hotspot item.

381. In the short-axis view of the great vessels, all of the following can be demonstrated EXCEPT the:
    A. Foramen ovale
    B. Pulmonic valve
    C. Left atrium
    D. Left ventricle
    E. Tricuspid valve

382. What is the best view to evaluate the number of aortic cusps?
    A. Apical four-chamber view
    B. Subcostal four-chamber view
    C. Long-axis view of the aorta
    D. Long-axis view of the pulmonary artery
    E. Short-axis view of the great vessels

383. The short-axis view of the ventricles can be used to help evaluate all of the following EXCEPT:
    A. Fetal arrhythmias
    B. Ventricular free wall thickness
    C. Interventricular septal defects
    D. Ventricular chamber diameter
    E. The moderator band

384. This image was taken in the following scan plane: *(See Color Plate 5 on page xix.)*

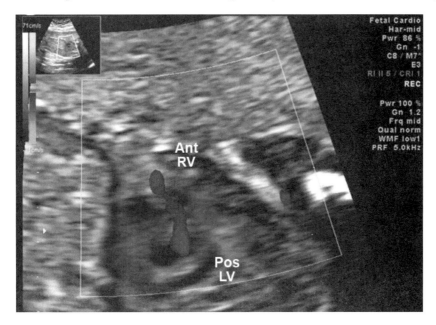

    A. Subcostal four-chamber view
    B. Short-axis view of the ventricles
    C. Long-axis view of the aorta
    D. Four-chamber view
    E. Five-chamber view

385. In the three-vessel view, which vessel is most anterior?
    A. Aorta
    B. Superior vena cava
    C. Pulmonary artery
    D. Ductus arteriosus
    E. Both A and C are at the same level.

386. What cardiac heart view was used to acquire this image?

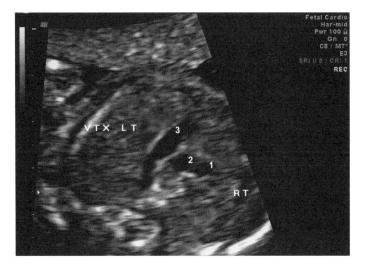

A. Long-axis view of the aorta

B. Three-vessel view

C. Short-axis view of the great arteries

D. Long-axis view of the pulmonary artery

E. Five-vessel view

387. Which of these statements about the ductus arteriosus is TRUE?

A. The ductus arteriosus has a "hockey stick" appearance.

B. The ductus arteriosus supplies blood to the fetal head and neck vessels.

C. The ductus arteriosus has a higher peak systolic velocity when compared to the aorta.

D. Both A and C are true.

E. Both A and B are true.

388. This image demonstrates a normal ductal arch view. All of the following should be visualized EXCEPT the:

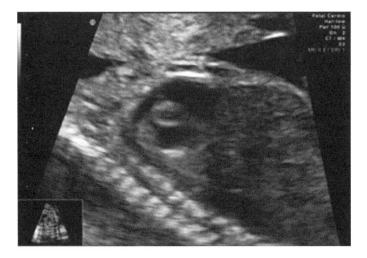

A. Mitral valve

B. Aortic valve

C. Pulmonic valve

    D. Tricuspid valve

    E. Ductus arteriosus

AIT—Hotspot item.

389. Which of these statements about evaluating the superior and inferior venae cavae is NOT true?

    A. The diameter of the superior vena cava is larger than that of the inferior vena cava.

    B. The diameter of the inferior vena cava is larger than that of the superior vena cava.

    C. Both the superior and inferior venae cavae flow into the right atrium.

    D. The inferior vena cava is seen to the right of the aorta in the fetal abdomen.

    E. The superior vena cava is seen coursing caudally entering the fetal heart.

390. This waveform (arrow) demonstrates:

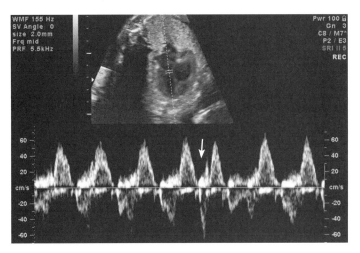

    A. Normal atrioventricular rate

    B. Premature atrial contraction

    C. Blocked premature atrial contraction

    D. Complete atrioventricular block

    E. Premature ventricular contraction

AIT—Hotspot item.

391. This waveform (arrow) demonstrates:

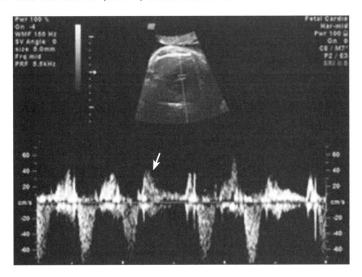

A. Normal atrioventricular rate

B. Premature atrial contraction

C. Blocked premature atrial contraction

D. Complete atrioventricular block

E. Premature ventricular contraction

AIT—Hotspot item.

392. What modality is used to display movements as they occur in tissue on a time axis?

A. B-mode

B. B-flow

C. Power Doppler

D. M-mode

E. Color Doppler imaging

393. Which of the following ultrasound modalities is used as a screening tool for cardiac activity in healthy pregnancies?

A. M-mode

B. B-mode

C. Pulsed-wave Doppler

D. Spectral Doppler

E. Color Doppler

394. What modality was used to obtain the fractional shortening percentile seen in this image?

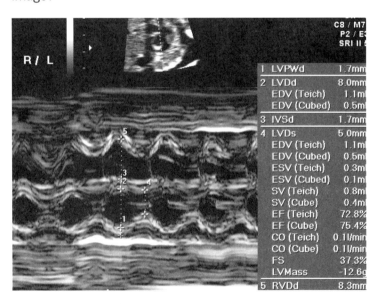

A. B-mode scanning

B. M-mode tracing

C. Pulsed-wave Doppler analysis

D. Color mode imaging

E. Spectral Doppler waveform

395. What heart view must be obtained to acquire an M-mode tracing that allows for measurement of the interventricular septal wall thickness and ventricular size?
    A. Short-axis view of the right ventricle
    B. Subcostal four-chamber view
    C. Three-vessel view
    D. Short-axis view of the left ventricle
    E. Both B and D are acceptable.

396. Which sonographic modality displays a single B-mode line of site along a horizontal axis?
    A. B-mode
    B. Pulsed-wave Doppler
    C. Spectral Doppler
    D. M-mode
    E. B-color

397. This M-mode image demonstrates that the heart rate of this second trimester fetus is:

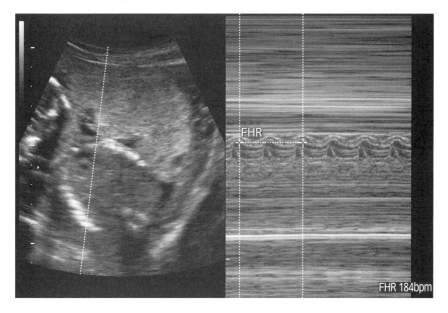

    A. Normal
    B. Irregular
    C. Tachycardic
    D. Bradycardic
    E. Blocked

398. The waveform below with the M-mode cursor passing through the left atrium and right ventricle demonstrates:

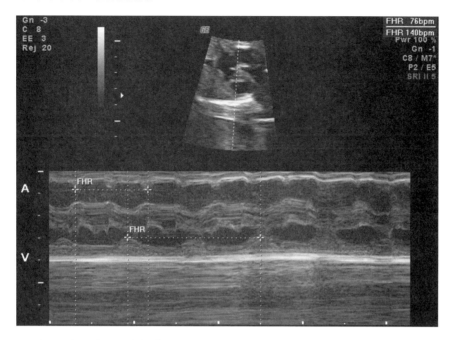

A. Complete heart block
B. Sinus bradycardia
C. Partial atrioventricular block
D. Supraventricular tachycardia
E. Premature atrial contractions

399. In this image the ratio of the cardiac circumference to the thoracic circumference (CC:TC ratio) was calculated. What CC:TC ratio is diagnostic of cardiomegaly?

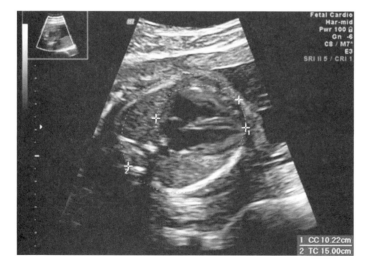

A. <0.3
B. <0.5
C. >0.5
D. <0.65
E. >0.75

400. In this image, a measurement was taken of a 28-week fetus in the vertex presentation. What are the calipers measuring, and would you assess this measurement of 0.63 cm to be normal or abnormal?

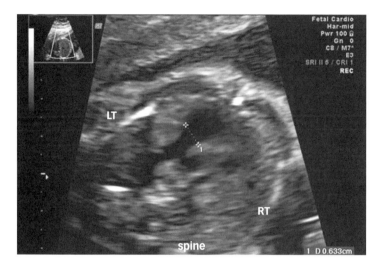

    A. Aortic valve; normal

    B. Aortic valve; abnormal

    C. Pulmonic valve; normal

    D. Pulmonic valve; abnormal

    E. Tricuspid valve; normal

AIT—Hotspot item.

401. When evaluating for an atrial septal defect, the examiner must know that the atrial-to-ventricular ratio in a normal fetus should be:

    A. 1:1

    B. 1:3

    C. 2:1

    D. 1:2

    E. 3:1

402. In this image the calipers are measuring:

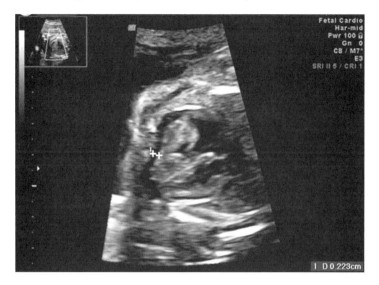

A. Pleural effusion

B. Pericardial effusion

C. Myocardium

D. Posterior ventricular wall

E. Pericardial fat

AIT—Hotspot item.

403. What would be considered a normal appearance and a normal amount of fluid around the fetal heart?

A. No evidence of fluid around the fetal heart

B. Hypoechoic rim of fluid less than 2 mm

C. Hypoechoic rim of fluid less than 3 mm

D. Hypoechoic rim of fluid less than 2 cm

E. Hypoechoic rim of fluid less than 3 cm

PART 6

Physics and Instrumentation

Imaging instruments

Adjust console settings to achieve optimal imaging display

Perform quality assurance checks on the equipment

Select the proper transducer

Artifacts

Modify the console settings based on color Doppler artifacts

Modify the console settings based on gray-scale artifacts

Modify the console settings based on spectral Doppler artifacts

Hemodynamics

Use color Doppler to assess blood flow

Use power Doppler to assess blood flow

Use pulsed-wave Doppler to assess blood flow

404. What is the most important physical parameter influencing absorption of the sound beam?
    A. Frequency
    B. Wall filter
    C. Reject
    D. Contrast
    E. Frame rate

405. Absorption of energy from attenuation of the ultrasound beam as it travels through tissues is highest in:
    A. Urine
    B. Amniotic fluid
    C. Blood
    D. Soft tissue
    E. Bone

406. What function control equalizes the ultrasound signals received from various depths and displays them with equal reflections?
    A. Wall filter
    B. Focal zone
    C. Pulse repetition frequency
    D. Time gain compensation
    E. Sample volume size
AIT—SIC item.

407. What function controls the number of ultrasound pulses transmitted per second and is dependent on depth of penetration and sample volume?
    A. Depth gain compensation
    B. Pulse repetition frequency (PRF)
    C. Overall gain
    D. Wall filter
    E. Edge enhancement
AIT—SIC item.

408. Why is it important to choose the correct sample volume size?
    A. A small sample volume allows simultaneous tracing of the vessel and its surrounding vessels.
    B. A small sample volume prevents interference from the blood flow in nearby vessels.
    C. A sample volume that is too small will not allow all parts of the flow to be encompassed.
    D. The sample volume should be adapted to fit the diameter of the vessel being interrogated.
    E. All of these statements are true except A.

409. For this image, what can you do to eliminate the poor visualization at the apex of the heart?

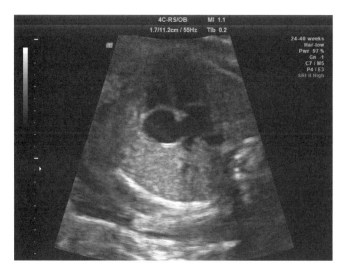

   A. Adjust the focal zone closer to the apex.
   B. Increase frequency.
   C. Decrease frequency.
   D. A and B.
   E. A and C.

AIT—SIC item.

410. In order to obtain the most precise image, the area of interest should be focused in what part of the sound beam?
   A. Near field
   B. Far field
   C. Divergent field
   D. Nyquist zone
   E. Frame path

411. Which phrase, commonly referred to as ALARA, signifies the clinical standard of practice regarding both the patient's and the examiner's exposure to acoustic output during an ultrasound exam?
   A. As long as [is] reasonably acceptable
   B. As low as [is] reasonably achievable
   C. All limits are regarded [as] acceptable
   D. All liable assistants [should] read and approve
   E. As low as [the] registered allowance

412. What term describes the reaction of gas bubbles in the patient's tissues resulting from the energy transmitted by the ultrasound beam?
   A. Cavitation
   B. Evaporation
   C. Condensation
   D. Reverberation
   E. Absorption

413. Which of these phenomena associated with the passage of the ultrasound beam through body tissues are classified as bioeffects (biological effects)?
     A. Thermal effects
     B. Transient effects
     C. Mechanical effects
     D. Reverberation effects
     E. A and C

414. The rise in temperature in tissues under the influence of ultrasound energy is controlled by the power level settings on the ultrasound machine. Which of the following is considered an INSIGNIFICANT rise in temperature?
     A. <1 degree Celsius
     B. <1.5 degrees Celsius
     C. <2.0 degrees Celsius
     D. <2.2 degrees Celsius
     E. No rise in temperature is safe.

415. Which of the following is the best description of the ALARA principle?
     A. Limiting exposure to gas-filled tissues
     B. Reducing the mechanical index to the lowest value consistent with effective imaging
     C. Keeping both output power and exposure time as low as reasonably achievable
     D. Reducing the thermal index to the lowest value consistent with effective imaging
     E. Scanning only the location needed for a complete consistent examination

416. Where does maximum tissue heating occur during an ultrasound exam?
     A. Between the transducer surface and the focal zone
     B. At the focal zone
     C. In the far field
     D. Between the focal zone and far field
     E. Throughout the entire width of the scan sector

417. The optimal transducer frequency for obstetric fetal echocardiography is:
     A. 2 MHz
     B. 3–5 MHz
     C. 5–7 MHz
     D. 8–10 MHz
     E. 12 MHz

418. The transducer emits a sound beam across the field of view. What term describes the location where the sound beam reaches its narrowest diameter?
     A. Near field
     B. Far field
     C. Focal zone
     D. Bandwidth
     E. Frame path

419. This ultrasound image was taken with the fetus in vertex presentation. What should be done to improve the quality of the image? *(See Color Plate 6 on page xix.)*

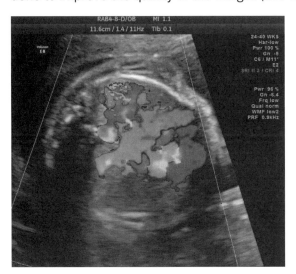

 A. Increase pulse repetition frequency (PRF)
 B. Decrease sample volume
 C. Decrease frame rate
 D. Decrease PRF
 E. Decrease penetration

AIT—SIC item.

420. What adjustments will eliminate aliasing?
 A. Changing the angle of insonation
 B. Shifting the baseline
 C. Lowering the frequency
 D. Increasing the pulse repetition frequency (PRF)
 E. All of the above

AIT—SIC item.

421. Shadowing occurs when the object of interrogation has a high level of:
 A. Absorption
 B. Attenuation
 C. Reflection
 D. Refraction
 E. Deflection

422. What artifact—caused by two strong reflectors with a large surface area—is displayed in the near field and has multiple, equally spaced echoes that extend into the far field?
 A. Bandwidth artifact
 B. Reverberation artifact
 C. Side-lobe artifact
 D. Mirror-image artifact
 E. Speckle artifact

AIT—Hotspot item.

423. Name the artifact observed in this image:

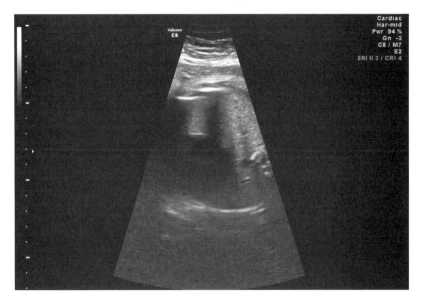

A. Comet-tail artifact

B. Shadowing

C. Aliasing

D. Mirror-image artifact

E. Crosstalk artifact

AIT—Hotspot item.

424. Which of the following is NOT true of shadowing artifacts?

A. They appear as hypoechoic or anechoic.

B. They are located beneath the structure with abnormally high attenuation.

C. They result from too much attenuation.

D. They represent multiple reflections of the same object.

E. They prevent visualization of true anatomy on the scan.

425. What can the sonographer do to eliminate the artifact seen in question 423?

A. Decrease the frequency.

B. Adjust angle of insonation to avoid scanning through fetal ribs.

C. Adjust the frame rate.

D. Adjust rejection.

E. All of these adjustments will eliminate this artifact.

AIT—SIC item.

426. What is causing the artifact seen in question 423?

A. Fetal rib shadows

B. Air bubbles under the surface of the transducer

C. A poor acoustic window

D. Fetal breathing movements

E. A and C

427. When scanning the fetal heart in the apical four-chamber view, the sonographer must be familiar with a common artifact that occurs near the crux of the heart. What is the name of this artifact, seen in this image?

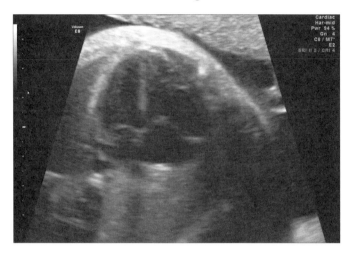

   A. Reverberation artifact
   B. Dropout artifact
   C. Edge-enhancement artifact
   D. Aliasing artifact
   E. Comet-tail artifact

AIT—Hotspot item.

428. What is causing the artifact in the image in question 427?
   A. The transmitted sound beam is perpendicular to the septum.
   B. The transmitted sound beam is parallel to the septum.
   C. The transmitted sound beam is attenuated by the fetal sternum.
   D. The transmitted sound beam is reflected by fetal breathing movements.
   E. The transmitted sound beam is deflected by the atrioventricular valve movements.

429. This image of the aortic arch has equally spaced, hypoechoic echoes projecting into the far field. What is this artifact called, and what is causing it?

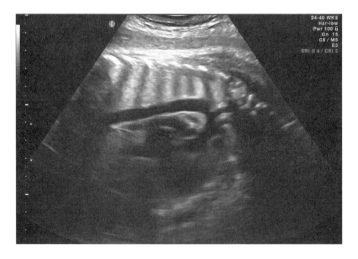

A. Bandwidth artifact caused by amniotic fluid

B. Bandwidth artifact caused by fetal ribs

C. Shadowing artifact caused by fetal ribs

D. Side-lobe artifact caused by increased maternal body habitus

E. Shadowing artifact caused by amniotic fluid

430. Which type of artifact is produced by interference patterns and results in the granular appearance of the image?

A. Speckle

B. Attenuation

C. Side-lobe artifact

D. Mirror-image artifact

E. Enhancement

431. What function is used to eliminate low-frequency noise and artifactual clutter caused by the movement of the vessel walls?

A. Time gain compensation

B. Edge enhancement

C. Pulse inversion

D. Wall filter

E. Baseline

AIT—SIC item.

432. The ultrasound flow velocity seen in this image was obtained across the tricuspid valve. What type of artifact is observed? *(See Color Plate 7 on page xx.)*

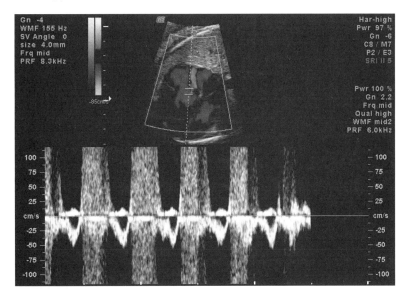

A. Aliasing

B. Side lobe

C. Speckle

D. Noise

E. Baseline shift

AIT—Hotspot item.

433. Which of the following adjustments will NOT optimize the image in question 432?
    A. Decreasing transducer frequency
    B. Increasing scale
    C. Increasing pulse repetition frequency
    D. Decreasing overall gain
    E. Decreasing the baseline

AIT—SIC item.

434. In this Doppler tracing of the umbilical artery, what setting needs to be adjusted? *(See Color Plate 8 on page xx.)*

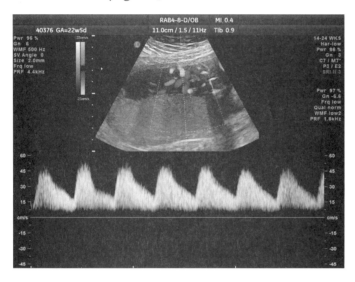

    A. Speed
    B. Pulse repetition frequency (PRF)
    C. Scale
    D. Frequency
    E. Wall filter

AIT—SIC item.

435. How should the controls be adjusted to decrease the noise in this spectral tracing of the ductus venosus? *(See Color Plate 9 on page xxi.)*

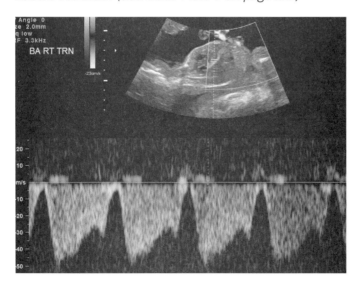

A. Increase overall gain.

B. Decrease overall gain.

C. Increase color gain.

D. Decrease color gain.

E. Increase wall filter.

AIT—SIC item.

436. What is the term for a frequency shift that exceeds the Nyquist limit during pulsed-wave or color Doppler imaging?

A. Reflection

B. Refraction

C. Compensation

D. Demodulation

E. Aliasing

437. The spectral Doppler tracing in this image is of the mitral valve/aortic valve. How should you adjust the parameters to optimize the tracing and evaluate the aortic peak velocity?

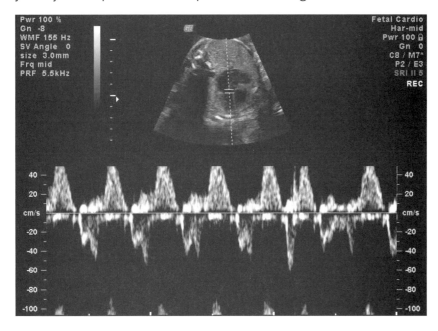

A. Decrease the sample volume gate.

B. Increase speed.

C. Adjust the baseline.

D. Use angle correction.

E. None of the above.

AIT—SIC item.

438. What Doppler mode was used to obtain this image? *(See Color Plate 10 on page xxi.)*

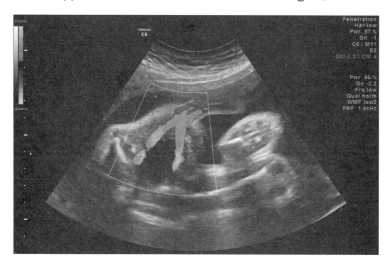

    A. Color Doppler imaging

    B. Power Doppler

    C. High-definition Doppler

    D. Continuous-wave Doppler

    E. M-mode Doppler

439. Color Doppler imaging gives information on:

    A. Blood flow velocity

    B. Blood flow direction

    C. Frequency shift

    D. Blood flow disturbances

    E. All of the above

440. Which of the following can be determined with the image in question 438?

    A. Blood flow velocity

    B. Blood flow direction

    C. Blood flow turbulence

    D. A and B only

    E. All of the above

441. This ultrasound image was obtained with the fetus in breech presentation, head to maternal right and spine down. The color Doppler spectrum demonstrates what type of flow pattern across the ductus arteriosus? *(See Color Plate 11 on page xxii.)*

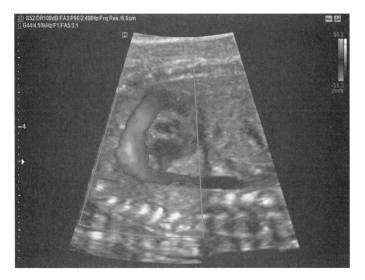

A. Reversed flow
B. Retrograde flow
C. Antegrade flow
D. Continuous flow
E. Both C and D

442. In this image the arrow is pointing to the ductus venosus. What does the variation of the color signal represent? *(See Color Plate 12 on page xxii.)*

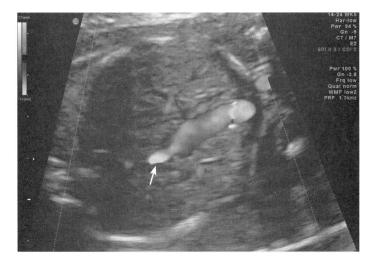

A. Continuous flow
B. Aliasing
C. Retrograde flow
D. Compression
E. Scatter

AIT—Hotspot item.

443. This is an image of a 28-week fetus in vertex presentation, spine up. The color spectrum displays which of the following? *(See Color Plate 13 on page xxiii.)*

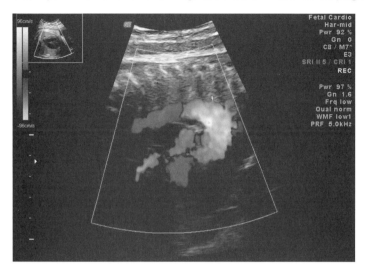

   A. Retrograde flow across the aortic arch
   B. Reversed flow across the aortic arch
   C. Bidirectional flow across the aortic arch
   D. Antegrade flow across the aortic arch
   E. Absent flow across the aortic arch

444. What Doppler mode was used to obtain the image in question 443?
   A. Power Doppler
   B. Color Doppler
   C. High-definition Doppler
   D. Continuous-wave Doppler
   E. M-mode Doppler

445. In this image, a large muscular ventricular septal defect is seen. How should the flow across the defect in this frame be interpreted? *(See Color Plate 14 on page xxiii.)*

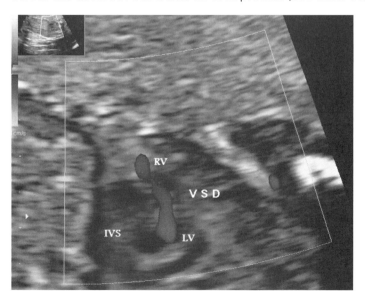

A. Flow is bidirectional across the defect.

B. Flow is from the right ventricle to the left ventricle.

C. Flow is from the left ventricle to the right ventricle.

D. The flow state cannot be determined from this image.

E. Flow is absent.

446. In order to visualize flow in vessels with low-flow states such as the pulmonary veins, what adjustment must the sonographer make?

A. Decrease the pulse repetition frequency (PRF).

B. Increase scale.

C. Decrease the color gain.

D. Both A and C.

E. Both B and C.

AIT—SIC item.

447. What Doppler mode was used to obtain this image? *(See Color Plate 15 on page xxiv.)*

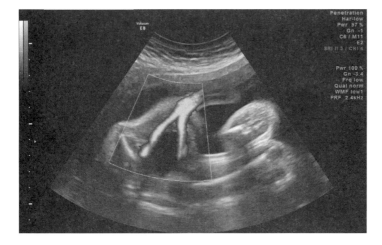

A. Color Doppler imaging

B. Power Doppler

C. High-definition Doppler

D. Continuous-wave Doppler

E. M-mode Doppler

448. What are the benefits of power Doppler compared to color Doppler?

A. Power Doppler is less dependent on the angle of incidence.

B. Power Doppler is not subject to aliasing.

C. Power Doppler is less dependent on direction of blood flow.

D. Power Doppler is useful in slow-flow velocity states.

E. All of the above are benefits.

449. Which of the following can be evaluated with the image in question 447?

A. Blood flow velocity

B. Blood flow direction

C. Blood flow turbulence

D. A and B only

E. None of the above

450. What functions are available when using power Doppler?
    A. Baseline
    B. Scale
    C. Pulse repetition frequency (PRF)
    D. Color gain
    E. None of these functions is available with power Doppler.

451. In a Doppler waveform across the mitral valve, the A wave represents:
    A. Early diastolic filling
    B. Early systolic filling
    C. Atrial systole
    D. Ventricular systole
    E. Late systole

452. Normal patent foramen ovale flow is:
    A. Monophasic, 20–40 cm/sec
    B. Monophasic, 50–70 cm/sec
    C. Biphasic, 20–40 cm/sec
    D. Biphasic, 50–70 cm/sec
    E. Triphasic, 20–40 cm/sec

453. Pulsatile flow in the umbilical vein seen with Doppler ultrasonography most likely represents:
    A. Normal Doppler flow pattern
    B. Congestive heart failure
    C. Volume overload
    D. Premature atrial contraction
    E. Both B and C

454. Which of the following can be determined from this spectral Doppler tracing of the ductus arteriosus?

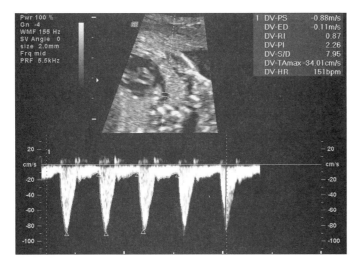

A. Peak systolic velocity

B. Pulsatility index

C. Resistivity index

D. Systolic/diastolic ratio

E. All of the above

455. This image is a pulsed-wave Doppler signal of the ductus venosus. What type of flow does the waveform represent? *(See Color Plate 16 on page xxiv.)*

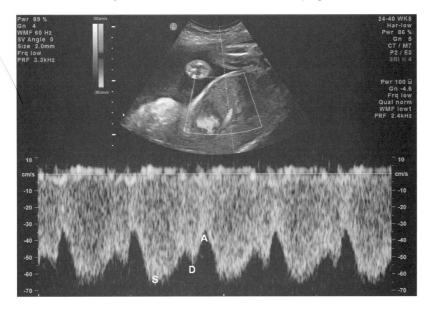

A. Monophasic flow

B. Biphasic flow

C. Triphasic flow

D. Retrograde flow

E. Absent end flow

456. What indices of the ductus venosus can you calculate based on the waveform in question 455?

A. Peak velocity in systole

B. Early diastole

C. Atrial contraction

D. Average maximum velocity

E. All of the above

457. If a fetus has a cardiac malformation with reduced cardiac inflow, the ductus venosus waveform will be abnormal. The abnormal waveform will have:

A. Reduced A wave toward the baseline

B. Reversed flow of the A wave during atrial contraction

C. Double pulsations in the waveform

D. Increased velocity of the S wave

E. Both A and B

458. When you are performing a pulsed-wave Doppler sample of the umbilical vein, it is important to avoid errors in the interpretation of an abnormal pulsatile waveform. Which of the following may cause erroneous samples?
    A. Umbilical arterial flow included in a large sample volume
    B. Fetal breathing movements
    C. Fetal hiccups
    D. Cord compression
    E. All of the above

Questions 459–461 refer to this image of a pulsed-wave Doppler signal obtained across the tricuspid valve, which demonstrates a biphasic flow pattern.

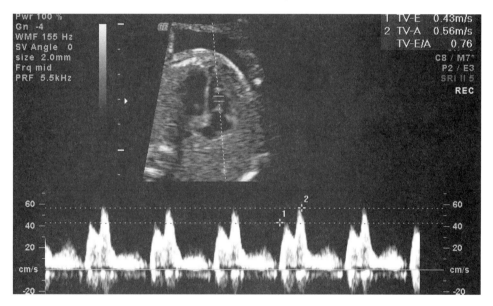

459. What is caliper 1 measuring?
    A. A wave
    B. B wave
    C. D wave
    D. E wave
    E. S wave
AIT—Hotspot item.

460. What is caliper 2 measuring?
    A. A wave
    B. B wave
    C. D wave
    D. E wave
    E. S wave
AIT—Hotspot item.

461. How did the sonographer manipulate parameters to obtain the E and A waves?
    A. By placing the sample volume gate distal to the tricuspid valve
    B. By maintaining the angle of insonation at 0 degrees
    C. By setting the sample volume size at 2 mm
    D. A and B
    E. A, B, and C

AIT—SIC item.

462. Which modality transmits the greatest amount of energy into the fetus?
    A. 2D imaging
    B. Pulsed-wave Doppler
    C. Color Doppler
    D. Power Doppler
    E. M-mode

463. Of the following velocities across the ductus arteriosus, which one would NOT be considered normal?
    A. >70 cm per second
    B. >84 cm per second
    C. >100 cm per second
    D. >120 cm per second
    E. >140 cm per second

PART 7

Managing Medical Emergencies

Assist patient experiencing a vasovagal response

Inform the supervising physician of findings of an emergent nature

464. What is most likely to cause a healthy patient to experience a warm, flushed feeling and nausea during an ultrasound examination in the supine position?
    A. Vasovagal response
    B. Poor ventilation in the ultrasound room
    C. Maternal fever
    D. Pressing too hard on the maternal abdomen with the transducer
    E. Maternal hyperthyroidism

465. Your third trimester patient feels faint and nauseated during the examination. What should you do?
    A. Roll her onto her left side, right side up.
    B. Administer smelling salts.
    C. Maintain her supine position and have her breathe deeply.
    D. Raise her head and have her sip water.
    E. Lower the head end of the examination table to place her in a Trendelenburg position.

466. You are measuring the fetal pole and there is no cardiac activity. Which length would indicate fetal demise?
    A. >2 mm
    B. >2 cm
    C. >5 mm
    D. >5 cm
    E. >10 cm

467. Diagnosis of a ductal-dependent heart lesion requires immediate reporting to the referring physician in order to prepare an appropriate delivery plan. All the following defects are ductal-dependent lesions EXCEPT:
    A. D-transposition of the great arteries
    B. L-transposition of the great arteries
    C. Hypoplastic left heart syndrome
    D. Coarctation of the aorta
    E. Severe pulmonic stenosis

468. What medical therapy is used to keep the ductus arteriosus patent postnatally?
    A. Digoxin
    B. Prostaglandin E
    C. Indomethacin
    D. Bradykinin
    E. Potassium

469. Ebstein anomaly is associated with several conditions. Which of the following makes close surveillance of this heart defect necessary?
    A. Tachyarrhythmia
    B. Hydrops fetalis
    C. Cardiomegaly
    D. Tricuspid dysplasia
    E. All these associated complications make close surveillance necessary.

470. Which of these dysrhythmias requires close surveillance because of its high association with structural heart defects and increased risk for hydrops?
    A. Complete heart block
    B. Premature atrial contraction
    C. Ventricular tachycardia
    D. Atrial bigeminy
    E. Premature ventricular contraction

471. A routine 30-week ultrasound reveals supraventricular tachycardia with no evidence of hydrops. Recommended treatment is:
    A. No treatment
    B. Another ultrasound exam in one week
    C. Maternal digoxin therapy
    D. Immediate delivery
    E. Fetal echocardiography at 28 weeks

472. A fetus whose routine 35-week ultrasound reveals supraventricular tachycardia develops hydrops and has poor fetal testing. The recommended treatment would be:
    A. No treatment
    B. Repeat ultrasound in one week
    C. Maternal digoxin therapy
    D. Immediate delivery
    E. Percutaneous umbilical cord blood sampling procedure

473. Twin-to-twin transfusion syndrome is associated with a higher risk for what fetal heart condition in the recipient twin?
    A. Hypertrophic cardiomyopathy
    B. Restrictive cardiomyopathy
    C. Dilated cardiomyopathy
    D. Endocardial fibroelastosis
    E. Hypoplasia of the left ventricle

474. A fetal echo exam is indicated for a fetus with pericardial effusions, which may be caused by high-output failure. Which of the following is considered to be a cause the effusion?
    A. Twin-to-twin transfusion syndrome
    B. Arteriovenous malformation
    C. Fetal anemias
    D. A and B
    E. All of the above

475. Which of these criteria must be met to consider treating a fetal cardiac anomaly prenatally?
    A. The lesion must have a poor prognosis with standard therapy.
    B. Fetal intervention will slow or halt progression of the lesion.
    C. The lesion cannot be treated postnatally.
    D. Both A and B.
    E. All of the above.

PART 8

Answers, Explanations, and References

PART 1

Anatomy and Physiology

1. A. Aorta.

2. C. 1/3 the diameter.

    The area of the aorta just distal to the left subclavian artery is the isthmus. *In the fetus and newborn, the aorta gradually becomes narrower, with the isthmus having the smallest diameter. In utero, the diameter of the isthmus is approximately two-thirds narrower than the diameter of the ascending and descending aorta. After birth, the isthmus enlarges once the ductus arteriosus closes.*

    ▶ Drose JA: *Fetal Echocardiography*, 2nd edition. St. Louis, Saunders Elsevier, 2010, p 190.

3. E. All of the above are true.

    The normal left aortic arch gives off an initial branch to the right, called the innominate *(also known as the* brachiocephalic*) artery. The innominate artery divides into the right subclavian and right common carotid arteries. The aortic arch curves over the right pulmonary artery.*

4. C. Left subclavian artery.

5. B. Left common carotid artery.

6. A. Innominate artery.

7. D. Right pulmonary artery.

8. B. Right ventricle.

9. C. Right ventricle.

    The right ventricle contains a moderator band near the apex of the heart. This moderator band gives the right ventricle a shorter lumen and its distinctive "trabecular" appearance.

    ▶ Yagel S, Silverman NH, Gembruch U: *Fetal Cardiology*. London, Martin Dunitz, 2003, pp 24–25.
    ▶ Yagel S, Silverman NH, Gembruch U: *Fetal Cardiology*. London, Informa Healthcare, 2008.

10. B. It contains the mitral valve.

    The mitral valve is a morphologic marker of the left ventricle, NOT *the left atrium.*

11. E. All of the above.

    The normal left ventricle has septophobic mitral valve attachments away from the septum, is smooth-walled, and has two papillary muscles; the mitral valve is located more superiorly than the tricuspid valve.

12. A. It has a finger-like, thin appendage.

    The left atrium has a finger-like, thin appendage. The right atrium has a broad-based appendage, contains the sinoatrial node, and receives the inferior and superior venae cavae.

13. E. Exhibits all of these characteristics.

    The normal right ventricle has a moderator band, is trabeculated, has septophilic attachments of the tricuspid valve, and is triangular in shape.

14. B. Right atrium.

15. C. Foramen ovale.

16. A. Left atrium.

17. C. Moderator band.

18. A. Right ventricle.

19. C. Tricuspid valve.

20. D. Right atrium.

21. B. Left ventricle.

22. D. Mitral valve.

23. C. Left atrium.

24. E. Pulmonary veins.

25. D. Foramen ovale.

26. E. All of these statements are true.

27. D. B (ductus arteriosus) and C (patent foramen ovale).

    There are three fetal shunts, including the ductus venosus, *which allows oxygenated blood flow from the umbilical vein to bypass the liver and enter directly into the inferior vena cava; the* ductus arteriosus, *which allows blood from the pulmonary trunk to bypass the lungs and shunt to into the aortic arch and descending aorta; and the* patent foramen ovale, *which allows oxygenated blood to flow from the right atrium to the left atrium. The ductus arteriosus and foramen ovale are the heart shunts. Since the fetus cannot use its own lungs to obtain oxygenated blood, these shunts make it possible for the maternal lungs to provide the fetus with oxygenated blood flow.*

28. A. Mitral valve.

29. C. 3 cusps.

30. B. Is continuous with the posterior wall of the aorta.

    The mitral valve can be seen in continuity with the aorta. The mitral valve contains only two leaflets and
    is located posterior and inferior to the tricuspid valve.

    ▸ Lai WW, Mertens LL, Cohen MS, et al: *Echocardiography in Pediatric and Congenital Heart Disease: From Fetus to Adult,*
    2nd edition. Hoboken, Wiley, 2016, p 531.

31. A. The aortic valve is to the right and posterior to the pulmonic valve.

    The two semilunar valves of the heart are the aortic and pulmonic valves.

32. E. Aortic valve.

33. A. Left atrium.

34. C. Left ventricle.

35. D. Right ventricle.

36. D. A (superior and inferior venae cavae) and B (coronary sinus).

    In a normal heart, the superior vena cava, inferior vena cava, and coronary sinus all drain into the right atrium, and the pulmonary veins drain into the left atrium.

37. A. Coronary sinus.

38. C. Apical four-chamber view.

39. A. Left coronary artery.

    The best view to evaluate the fetal coronary sinus is the apical four-chamber view, directed posteriorly through the atria.

40. E. Left coronary artery.

41. B. Superior vena cava.

42. A. Aorta.

43. D. Main pulmonary artery.

44. C. The pulmonary artery, ductus arteriosus, and descending aorta.

45. D. Ductus arteriosus.

46. D. Stomach.

47. C. Left upper abdomen below the diaphragm.

48. E. All the above.

    The spleen, liver, aorta, and inferior vena cava (IVC) must all be evaluated to rule out abnormal fetal situs, which is commonly related to left and right atrial isomerism. In the presence of atrial isomerism, an abnormal arrangement of the liver and spleen may be noted. The spleen may be absent or multiple. The aorta must be evaluated for its relationship to the IVC, and the IVC can be transposed or interrupted.

49. D. Three-vessel view.

    The trachea is seen as a hypoechoic circle with an echogenic wall on the right side of the aorta and behind the superior vena cava in the three-vessel view. The position of the trachea is a landmark to distinguish the correct left-sided aortic arch from an abnormal right-sided aortic arch. Refer to questions 63–66.

    ▶ Yagel S, Silverman NH, Gembruch U: *Fetal Cardiology*. London, Martin Dunitz, 2003, pp 148–149.

    ▶ Yagel S, Silverman NH, Gembruch U: *Fetal Cardiology*. London, Informa Healthcare, 2008.

50. C. <33%.

    The normal heart occupies less than one-third of the fetal chest, i.e., 33% of the area of the thoracic cavity. If the heart area measures more than 33% of the area of the fetal thorax cavity, this would be considered cardiomegaly.

51. D. A (the esophagus appears as a tubular echogenic structure with a pattern of two echogenic lines) and C (the size of the esophagus varies with fetal swallowing).

    The fetal esophagus is an echogenic tubular structure that is visualized as two echogenic lines in the fetal neck and thorax. These lines may have a multilayered pattern. Fetal swallowing may be seen intermittently. The fetal esophagus will show variation in size during the examination; the trachea does not show a size change. The trachea is anterior to the esophagus and bifurcates into the main bronchi, while the esophagus continues without division.

    ▶ Avni WF, Rypens F, Milaire J: Fetal esophagus: normal sonographic appearance. J Ultrasound Med 13:175–180, 1994.

52. A. Establish fetal position.

A fetal echocardiography examination involves a sequential segmental analysis, which the sonographer must follow for every examination. First establishing the fetal position—either vertex breech or transverse lie—will allow one to determine fetal right and left sides. The segmental analysis includes an initial assessment of fetal right/left orientation, followed by an assessment of visceral/abdominal situs, stomach position, and cardiac apex position.

▶ American Institute of Ultrasound in Medicine: AIUM practice parameter for the performance of fetal echocardiography. AIUM, 2013, p 3. Available at http://www.aium.org/resources/guidelines/fetalecho.pdf.

▶ Drose JA: *Fetal Echocardiography*, 2nd edition. St. Louis, Saunders Elsevier, 2010, p 27.

53. B. Identify the location and orientation of the heart apex.

Following assessment of fetal position and right/left orientation as the initial steps in the segmental analysis, the next steps are to assess cardiac apex position along with visceral/abdominal situs and stomach position.

▶ American Institute of Ultrasound in Medicine: AIUM practice parameter for the performance of fetal echocardiography. AIUM, 2013, p 3. Available at http://www.aium.org/resources/guidelines/fetalecho.pdf.

▶ Drose JA: *Fetal Echocardiography*, 2nd edition. St. Louis, Saunders Elsevier, 2010, pp 27–28.

54. C. Dextroposition.

Dextroposition is an abnormal heart position, with the heart in the right chest and the apex pointing left.

▶ Drose JA: *Fetal Echocardiography*, 2nd edition. St. Louis, Saunders Elsevier, 2010, p 27.

55. A. 20 degrees.

The normal heart angle relative to midline is 45 degrees (± 20 degrees). The line traversing the interventricular septum and a line coursing from spine to mid chest should intersect at an angle of 25 to 65 degrees. This correct angle is normal levoposition of the fetal heart.

▶ Drose JA: *Fetal Echocardiography*, 2nd edition. St. Louis, Saunders Elsevier, 2010, pp 27, 74.

56. B. Levocardia.

Normal heart position in the fetal thorax is termed levocardia. *The normal heart is situated in the left chest with the apex pointing to the left. The axis of the heart relative to midline should be 45 degrees (± 20 degrees).*

57. D. Levocardia.

Normal heart position in the fetal thorax is termed levocardia. *The normal heart is situated in the left chest with the apex pointing to the left. The axis of the heart should be 45 degrees (± 20 degrees). In this image the fetus is in vertex presentation, the left side would be down, and the axis is normal. This image demonstrates normal levocardia.*

58. D. Main pulmonary artery.

59. A. Pulmonary veins.

60. E. All of the statements above are true.

The pulmonic valve lies anterior and superior to the aortic valve.

61. D. 4.

In the normal fetal heart four separate pulmonary veins are seen entering the left atrium: the right upper, right lower, left upper, and left lower pulmonary veins.

62. A. Courses superior to the left bronchus.

The normal left pulmonary artery courses above (superior to) the left bronchus and runs more superiorly than the left pulmonary artery. The right pulmonary artery courses below (inferior to) the right bronchus and underneath the aortic arch.

63. D. Trachea.

64. B. Pulmonary artery.

65. A. Aorta.

66. D. Ductus arteriosus.

67. D. Patent ductus arteriosus.

68. C. Right pulmonary artery.

69. A. Pulmonic valve.

70. D. Main pulmonary artery.

71. C. Inferior vena cava.

    The inferior vena cava (IVC) is the vessel seen coursing through the fetal abdomen alongside the aorta. The IVC is to the fetal right and posterior to the aorta, just anterior to the fetal spine. The aorta and IVC must be evaluated in their entirety to rule out interruption.

72. A. Ductus venosus.

    The ductus venosus allows the majority of the blood flow to be shunted away from the liver. This blood then enters the heart via the inferior vena cava.

73. E. Both B (Eustachian valve) and C (Chiari network).

    Multiple echoes within the right atrium can represent the Eustachian valve (valve of the inferior vena cava) and/or the Chiari network. The Chiari network is a reticular network of fibers originating from the Eustachian valve and connecting to different parts of the right atrium.

74. D. Sinoatrial node.

    Rhythmic beating and heart contractions originate in the sinoatrial node, which lies in the right atrium of the heart. The sinoatrial node is also known as the nodus sinuatrialis, sinuatrial node, sinus node, *and* cardiac pacemaker.

    ▸ Drose JA: *Fetal Echocardiography*, 2nd edition. St. Louis, Saunders Elsevier, 2010, pp 2, 8.

    ▸ Hess DB, Hess LW: *Fetal Echocardiography*, 1st edition. New York, McGraw-Hill, 1998, p 12.

75. C. Increases with advancing pregnancy.

76. A. 0.5–1.0.

    The E wave increases from 25 cm/sec at 16 weeks' gestation to 45 cm/sec at term. The A wave remains constant throughout the pregnancy at approximately 45 cm/sec.

    ▸ Allan L, Hornberger L, Sharland G: *Textbook of Fetal Cardiology*. London, Greenwich Medical Media, 2000, p 85.

77. D. 100–180 beats per minute.

    ▸ Drose JA: *Fetal Echocardiography*, 2nd edition. St. Louis, Saunders Elsevier, 2010, p 306.

78. B. Fetal heart rate remains constant throughout gestation.

    The fetal heart rate changes throughout gestation. The rate initially is slow, increasing to approximately 177 beats per minute (bpm) at day 63, then decreasing to an average of 147 bpm by week 15. The heart rate will range between 100 and 180 bpm throughout the remainder of the pregnancy.

    ▸ Drose JA: *Fetal Echocardiography*, 2nd edition. St. Louis, Saunders Elsevier, 2010, p 306.

    ▸ Moore KL, Persaud TVN: *The Developing Human*, 9th edition. Philadelphia, Saunders Elsevier, 2013, p 290.

79. E. In the placenta.

Fetal gas exchange takes place in the placenta. Blood needs to return to the placenta for oxygenation.

▶ Drose JA: *Fetal Echocardiography*, 2nd edition. St. Louis, Saunders Elsevier, 2010, p 8.

80. C. Is in parallel.

Both the right and left ventricles eject in parallel into the systemic circulation for the fetus.

▶ Drose JA: *Fetal Echocardiography*, 2nd edition. St. Louis, Saunders Elsevier, 2010, p 8.

81. E. All of the above.

The normal patent ductus arteriosus shunts blood right to left from the pulmonary artery to the aorta, may be constricted with indomethacin (Indocin), and has a pulsatility index of 1.9–3.0.

82. A. Ductus venosus.

Once the blood enters the fetus via the umbilical vein, the majority of flow goes through the ductus venosus. There is a sphincter located at the level of the umbilical vein and ductus venosus that regulates the amount of blood flow to the liver. In order to prevent sudden overload of flow to the heart, the sphincter closes when the venous return is too high.

▶ Drose JA: *Fetal Echocardiography*, 2nd edition. St. Louis, Saunders Elsevier, 2010, pp 8.

83. D. Patent foramen ovale.

▶ Drose JA: *Fetal Echocardiography*, 2nd edition. St. Louis, Saunders Elsevier, 2010, pp 8–10.

84. B. Bradykinin.

▶ Drose JA: *Fetal Echocardiography*, 2nd edition. St. Louis, Saunders Elsevier, 2010, p 10.

85. B. Inferior vena cava.

The ductus venosus comes off the umbilical vein and connects to the inferior vena cava, which connects to the heart.

▶ Drose JA: *Fetal Echocardiography*, 2nd edition. St. Louis, Saunders Elsevier, 2010, pp 8–10.

86. E. All of the above are correct.

▶ Drose JA: *Fetal Echocardiography*, 2nd edition. St. Louis, Saunders Elsevier, 2010, pp 8–10.

87. C. Right ventricle.

The right ventricle ejects approximately two-thirds of the total ventricular cardiac output. Most of the output is through the ductus arteriosus.

▶ Drose JA: *Fetal Echocardiography*, 2nd edition. St. Louis, Saunders Elsevier, 2010, p 10.

88. D. 85%.

▶ Drose JA: *Fetal Echocardiography*, 2nd edition. St. Louis, Saunders Elsevier, 2010, pp 8–10.

89. A. 58%.

Blood flows out of the fetus via the umbilical arteries to the placenta, with an oxygen saturation of 58%.

▶ Drose JA: *Fetal Echocardiography*, 2nd edition. St. Louis, Saunders Elsevier, 2010, pp 8–10.

90. E. Pulmonary veins.

91. C. Definitive aorta.

During embryologic development six pairs of arteries known as the aortic arches arise from the truncus arteriosus. The left arch of the fourth pair and the common dorsal aorta become the definitive aorta, while the fourth right arch becomes the proximal portion of the right subclavian artery.

> Drose JA: *Fetal Echocardiography*, 2nd edition. St. Louis, Saunders Elsevier, 2010, pp 6–7.

92. B. Corrected transposition of the great arteries.

Abnormal looping of the heart tube to the left instead of the right results in ventricular inversion, which is known as corrected transposition of the great arteries (l-ventricular loop).

> Drose JA: *Fetal Echocardiography*, 2nd edition. St. Louis, Saunders Elsevier, 2010, p 12.

93. C. 21–28 days.

At approximately 28 days' gestation (typically between days 22 and 23), or by the end of the fourth week following conception, the fetal heart contractions begin. This occurs in the ventriculobulbar portion of the heart.

> Drose JA: *Fetal Echocardiography*, 2nd edition. St. Louis, Saunders Elsevier, 2010, pp 2–3.

> Moore KL, Persaud TVN: *The Developing Human*, 9th edition. Philadelphia, Saunders Elsevier, 2013, p 290.

94. B. Semilunar valves.

The development of the semilunar valves—the aortic valve and the pulmonic (pulmonary) valve—is completed by 9 weeks' gestation. The heart valves are the last structures to develop embryologically.

> Larsen WJ: *Human Embryology*, 2nd edition. Philadelphia, Saunders, 1997, pp 152, 173.

> Schoenwolf GC, Bleyl SB, Brauer BS, et al: *Larsen's Human Embryology*, 4th edition. New York, Churchill Livingstone Elsevier, 2008.

95. C. 8.

96. D. Left atrium.

Initially, there is a common pulmonary vein and a right and left pulmonary vein. All of these veins are absorbed, resulting in four pulmonary veins that enter into the left atrium. They are the right upper, right lower, left upper, and left lower pulmonary veins.

> Drose JA: *Fetal Echocardiography*, 2nd edition. St. Louis, Saunders Elsevier, 2010, pp 6–7.

97. E. All of the above.

The endocardial cushions are developed from the extracellular matrix. As illustrated here, the endocardial cushions (EC) grow outward and upward, fusing with the septum primum (SP) that descends from above and with the interventricular septum (IS) that rises from below to become the atrioventricular partitions. The endocardial cushions are involved in the formation of the semilunar (aortic and pulmonic) valves, atrioventricular valves, and membranous septum. Endocardial cushion abnormalities commonly result in atrioventricular valve canal defects. RA = right atrium, LA = left atrium, RV = right ventricle, LV = left ventricle.

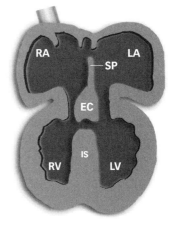

> Baun J: *Ob/Gyn Sonography: An Illustrated Review*. Pasadena, CA, Davies Publishing, 2016, p 157.

> Drose JA: *Fetal Echocardiography*, 2nd edition. St. Louis, Saunders Elsevier, 2010, pp 11–12.

> Moore KL, Persaud TVN: *The Developing Human*, 9th edition. Philadelphia, Saunders Elsevier, 2013, pp 299–300.

98. **E. All of the above.**

    Asplenia *and* polysplenia syndromes *are anomalies caused by a midline developmental field defect. This defect results in complex malformations of the abdominal and cardiovascular systems. Symmetry of these organ systems is affected.* Ivemark syndrome *and* right atrial isomerism *are both alternate terms for* asplenia.

    ▸ Drose JA: *Fetal Echocardiography*, 2nd edition. St. Louis, Saunders Elsevier, 2010, pp 281–282.

99. **C. 4 and 8.**

    All major organ systems are formed between 4 and 8 weeks' gestation. This time period is referred to as organogenesis. *Any factors that interfere with development of these organ systems may cause faulty development.*

    ▸ Drose JA: *Fetal Echocardiography*, 2nd edition. St. Louis, Saunders Elsevier, 2010, p 1.

100. **A. A normal great artery relationship (d-ventricular loop).**

    In normal fetal heart development, the heart tube bends slightly to the right, resulting in a normal relationship of the great arteries.

    ▸ Drose JA: *Fetal Echocardiography*, 2nd edition. St. Louis, Saunders Elsevier, 2010, p 12.

101. **E. Day 28.**

    ▸ Drose JA: *Fetal Echocardiography*, 2nd edition. St. Louis, Saunders Elsevier, 2010, p 105.

102. **E. All of the above.**

    Coarctation of the aorta (arrow) refers to a narrowing of the aortic lumen that results in reduced blood flow into the aortic arch. Signs include arch hypoplasia and diffuse narrowing of the aorta proximal to the ductus arteriosus. SVC = superior vena cava, DA = ductus arteriosus, RA = right atrium, LA = left atrium, RV = right ventricle, LV = left ventricle.

    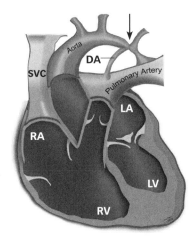

    ▸ Baun J: *Ob/Gyn Sonography: An Illustrated Review*. Pasadena, CA, Davies Publishing, 2016, p 185.

    ▸ Drose JA: *Fetal Echocardiography*, 2nd edition. St. Louis, Saunders Elsevier, 2010, pp 184–196.

    ▸ Moore KL, Persaud TVN: *The Developing Human*, 9th edition. Philadelphia, Saunders Elsevier, 2013, p 327.

103. **C. At 18–22 weeks' gestation.**

    The American Institute of Ultrasound in Medicine (AIUM) notes that for optimal visualization of the cardiac structures and for best image quality, a fetal echocardiographic exam is commonly performed between 18 and 22 weeks' gestation. At this time the fetus is large enough to evaluate the heart, but gestation is not yet advanced to the point where the study can encounter impeding factors, although AIUM notes that "some forms of congenital heart disease may … be recognized during earlier stages of pregnancy."

    ▸ American Institute of Ultrasound in Medicine: AIUM practice parameter for the performance of fetal echocardiography. AIUM, 2013. Available at http://www.aium.org/resources/guidelines/fetalecho.pdf.

    ▸ Drose JA: *Fetal Echocardiography*, 2nd edition. St. Louis, Saunders Elsevier, 2010, pp 16, 324.

    ▸ Lee W, Allan L, Carvalho JS, et al: ISUOG consensus statement: what constitutes a fetal echocardiogram? Ultrasound Obstet Gynecol 32:239–242, 2008.

104. **D. 11–16 weeks' gestation.**

    Several studies report that fetal echocardiography can be performed transvaginally as early as 11–16 weeks' gestation. Before 10 weeks' gestation the fetal heart is not fully developed and is generally too small to visualize the cardiac structures. Although there is some interest in first trimester echocardiography, it can be performed only as an adjunct to, not a replacement for, later studies.

    ▸ Drose JA: *Fetal Echocardiography*, 2nd edition. St. Louis, Saunders Elsevier, 2010, p 325.

PART 2
Pathology

105. A. Sinus tachycardia.

Sinus tachycardia is a heart rate greater than 180 beats per minute (bpm), with normal atrial and ventricular activation. Sinus tachycardia may have a variable heart rate. This dysrhythmia is usually brought on by an abnormal maternal or fetal condition, commonly maternal stress or fever.

▶ Drose JA: *Fetal Echocardiography*, 2nd edition. St. Louis, Saunders Elsevier, 2010, p 308.

106. B. Fluid seen in two or more fetal body cavities.

Fetal hydrops (or hydrops fetalis) is the excessive accumulation of fluid in at least two locations within the fetus. It is characterized by diffuse interstitial edema (anasarca), pleural and/or pericardial effusions, and ascites resulting from prenatal cardiac failure. The pathophysiologic problem is an imbalance in fluid homeostasis whereby more fluid is produced than is resorbed by normal physiologic processes. There are two types of hydrops fetalis: immune *(caused mainly by alloimmune hemolytic disease and Rh isoimmunization) and* nonimmune *(the result of a pathologic condition that disrupts the normal homeostatic mechanisms that control the fetal body's ability to manage fluid). Nonimmune hydrops is most commonly the result of fetal cardiovascular disease (25% of cases), including cardiac lesions, arrhythmias, and tumor-related high-output failure. Chromosomal anomalies account for 10% of nonimmune hydrops cases, thoracic lesions for 9%, twin-to-twin transfusion syndrome for 8%, fetal anemia for 6%, and fetal infection for 4%. See also answer 325.*

▶ Baun J: *Ob/Gyn Sonography: An Illustrated Review*. Pasadena, CA, Davies Publishing, 2016, pp 302–303.

▶ Callen PW: *Ultrasonography in Obstetrics and Gynecology*, 5th edition. Philadelphia, Saunders Elsevier, p 688.

107. B. 2%.

Cardiomyopathies account for approximately 2% of all cases of heart disease in live-born patients. There are three different presentations in the infant: congestive (dilated), hypertrophic, and restrictive.

▶ Drose JA: *Fetal Echocardiography*, 2nd edition. St. Louis, Saunders Elsevier, 2010, p 293.

108. E. 0.30.

The shortening fraction (SF) is useful in assessing poor heart function in cases of cardiomyopathy. Poor systolic function of the right and left ventricles will help in the assessment of the progression or resolution of the condition. Normal SF of the left ventricle is 0.30; normal SF of the right ventricle is 0.25.

SF = (EDD − ESD) / EDD

Abbreviations: SF = shortening fraction, EDD = end diastolic dimension, ESD = end systolic dimension.

▶ Drose JA: *Fetal Echocardiography*, 2nd edition. St. Louis, Saunders Elsevier, 2010, p 300.

109. C. Restrictive.

▶ Drose JA: *Fetal Echocardiography*, 2nd edition. St. Louis, Saunders Elsevier, 2010, pp 297–298.

110. A. Fetal anemias.

Fetal anemias are associated with dilated cardiomyopathy caused by high-output failure and poor cardiac function. Maternal diabetes, Noonan syndrome, glycogen storage disease, and twin-to-twin transfusion syndrome are associated with the hypertrophic form of cardiomyopathy.

▶ Drose JA: *Fetal Echocardiography*, 2nd edition. St. Louis, Saunders Elsevier, 2010, p 294.

111. E. C (congestive) and D (dilated).

Congestive cardiomyopathy, *also known as* dilated cardiomyopathy, *is the most common type.*

▸ Drose JA: *Fetal Echocardiography*, 2nd edition. St. Louis, Saunders Elsevier, 2010, p 293.

112. A. Maternal diabetes.

Poorly controlled maternal diabetes increases the risk for acquiring asymmetric septal hypertrophy or concentric hypertrophy of the left ventricle. The heart walls and septum may be thick.

▸ Drose JA: *Fetal Echocardiography*, 2nd edition. St. Louis, Saunders Elsevier, 2010, pp 296–297.

113. C. Hypertrophic cardiomyopathy.

The heart in this image appears thickened. In cases of hypertrophic cardiomyopathy, the ventricular walls and septum are grossly thickened.

▸ Drose JA: *Fetal Echocardiography*, 2nd edition. St. Louis, Saunders Elsevier, 2010, pp 296–298.

114. C. Short-axis view of the ventricles.

To observe fetal arrhythmias, the atrial and ventricular activity must be examined simultaneously. The short-axis view of the ventricles does NOT *image the atria.*

115. E. Polysplenia syndrome.

▸ Drose JA: *Fetal Echocardiography*, 2nd edition. St. Louis, Saunders Elsevier, 2010, pp 281–282.

116. B. Supraventricular tachycardia.

▸ Allan L, Hornberger L, Sharland G: *Textbook of Fetal Cardiology*. London, Greenwich Medical Media, 2000, pp 6–42.

117. E. A (bradycardia), B (complete heart block), and C (supraventricular tachycardia).

Cardiomyopathies may be associated with a dysrhythmia. The type and severity of the dysrhythmia depend on the cardiomyopathy and the underlying condition.

118. B. Atrial bigeminy.

Atrial bigeminy occurs when every other atrial contraction is premature and is not conducted to the ventricle.

▸ Drose JA: *Fetal Echocardiography*, 2nd edition. St. Louis, Saunders Elsevier, 2010, pp 308, 311.

119. A. Blocked premature atrial contraction.

▸ Drose JA: *Fetal Echocardiography*, 2nd edition. St. Louis, Saunders Elsevier, 2010, pp 309–311.

120. B. Premature atrial contractions.

Premature atrial contractions (PACs) are the most common dysrhythmia, secondary to isolated extrasystoles or premature beats. PACs are more common than premature ventricular contractions (PVCs).

▸ Drose JA: *Fetal Echocardiography*, 2nd edition. St. Louis, Saunders Elsevier, 2010, p 307.

121. B. Atrial flutter.

▸ Drose JA: *Fetal Echocardiography*, 2nd edition. St. Louis, Saunders Elsevier, 2010, p 308.

122. C. Sinus tachycardia.

Sinus tachycardia is a heart rate greater than 180 beats per minute (bpm) with normal atrial and ventricular activation.

▸ Drose JA: *Fetal Echocardiography*, 2nd edition. St. Louis, Saunders Elsevier, 2010, p 308.

123. **D. Nonconducted premature atrial contraction.**

Nonconducted premature atrial contraction *is an early atrial contraction. It is* NOT *followed by a ventricular contraction. A compensatory pause occurs, followed by normal sinus rhythm.*

▶ Woodward PJ, Kennedy A, Sohaey R, et al: *Diagnostic Imaging: Obstetrics.* Salt Lake City, AMIRSYS, 2005, ch 6, p 70.

124. **D. Supraventricular tachycardia.**

Fetal tachycardias are the second most common dysrhythmia, with supraventricular tachycardia occurring in 65% of cases. Sinus tachycardia is the most common tachycardia in general.

▶ Drose JA: *Fetal Echocardiography*, 2nd edition. St. Louis, Saunders Elsevier, 2010, p 308.

125. **B. Complete heart block.**

Complete heart block (third-degree heart block) is present when there is dissociation between the atrial and ventricular complexes. The atrial rate is faster than the ventricular rate.

▶ Drose JA: *Fetal Echocardiography*, 2nd edition. St. Louis, Saunders Elsevier, 2010, pp 308–309.

126. **E. Both A (second-degree heart block) and B (third-degree heart block [complete heart block]).**

Second- and third-degree heart block account for 96% of all bradycardias.

▶ Drose JA: *Fetal Echocardiography*, 1st edition. St. Louis, Saunders Elsevier, 1998, p 280.

127. **E. All of the above.**

Atrial fibrillation *is defined as an atrial rate of 300–500 beats per minute (bpm), with varying ventricular response. The ventricular rate may be fixed and regular, or variable and irregular.*

▶ Drose JA: *Fetal Echocardiography*, 2nd edition. St. Louis, Saunders Elsevier, 2010, p 308.

128. **D. L-transposition of the great arteries.**

In transposition of the great arteries *(TGA, also known as* transposition of the great vessels*), the pulmonary trunk arises from the left ventricle and the aorta arises from the right ventricle. There are two types:* complete TGA *or* dextrotransposition *(d-TGA) and* congenitally corrected TGA *or* levotransposition *(l-TGA). D-TGA accounts for approximately 80% of cases and if left untreated is lethal postnatally. Corrected transposition (l-TGA) is not lethal and is not considered a progressive lesion, although patients with this condition are at increased risk for heart failure as systemic right ventricular function declines with age. SVC = superior vena cava, RA = right atrium, LA = left atrium, RV = right ventricle, LV = left ventricle.*

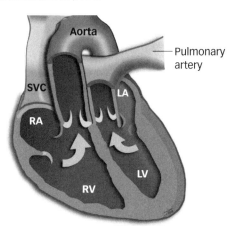

▶ Baun J: *Ob/Gyn Sonography: An Illustrated Review.* Pasadena, CA, Davies Publishing, 2016, p 177.

129. **A. Valvular aortic stenosis.**

Valvular aortic stenosis is the most common type of aortic stenosis, accounting for 60%–75% of cases.

▶ Drose JA: *Fetal Echocardiography*, 2nd edition. St. Louis, Saunders Elsevier, 2010, pp 169–170.

130. **D. Aortic valve stenosis.**

The prognosis for aortic stenosis depends on the severity of the lesion. When aortic stenosis is diagnosed in utero, the diagnosis is usually severe. If the pediatric patient is left untreated, endocardial fibroelastosis, small left heart, mitral stenosis, and small aorta will progress, and death commonly occurs.

▶ Drose JA: *Fetal Echocardiography*, 2nd edition. St. Louis, Saunders Elsevier, 2010, p 169.

131. B. E-wave mitral valve.

    The E wave is the "early" atrial filling of the mitral valve. See answer 460.

132. C. Mild to moderate pulmonary stenosis.

133. E. A (apical long-axis view of the pulmonary artery) and D (short-axis view of the great vessels).

134. D. Abnormal intracardiac blood flow.

    ▶ Drose JA: *Fetal Echocardiography*, 2nd edition. St. Louis, Saunders Elsevier, 2010, p 11.

135. A. Valvular pulmonic stenosis.

    Pulmonic stenosis most commonly occurs at the level of the pulmonic valve as a result of a defect in the valve. Various degrees of obstruction at this level may occur.

    ▶ Drose JA: *Fetal Echocardiography*, 2nd edition. St. Louis, Saunders Elsevier, 2010, pp 174–179.

136. D. Pulmonic stenosis.

    In cases of double-outlet right ventricle *(DORV), the aorta and the pulmonary artery both arise from the right ventricle. Other cardiac anomalies are usually present, including pulmonic stenosis approximately 70% of the time. SVC = superior vena cava, RA = right atrium, LA = left atrium, RV = right ventricle, LV = left ventricle, arrows = direction of blood flow.*

    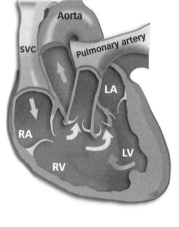

    ▶ Baun J: *Ob/Gyn Sonography: An Illustrated Review*. Pasadena, CA, Davies Publishing, 2016, p 180.

    ▶ Drose JA: *Fetal Echocardiography*, 2nd edition. St. Louis, Saunders Elsevier, 2010, pp 163.

137. C. Complete agenesis of the tricuspid valve.

138. D. A (ventricular septal defects), B (pulmonary atresia/stenosis), and C (hypoplasia of the right ventricle).

    Tricuspid atresia is the failure of the tricuspid valve and right ventricular inlet to form, resulting in a lack of direct communication between the right atrium and the right ventricle (white arrow). In the fetus, venous blood returning to the right atrium can cross the foramen ovale into the left heart, where the increased volume and pressure can cause volume overload. Some blood will reach the lungs through the ductus arteriosus, but the normal postnatal regression of this shunt presents the risk of serious complications. Accompanying anomalies may include atrial septal defect (arrow in the RA), ventricular septal defect (arrow entering the RV), right-sided aortic arch, transposition of the great vessels, and pulmonary atresia/stenosis. SVC = superior vena cava, RA = right atrium, LA = left atrium, RV = right ventricle, LV = left ventricle.

    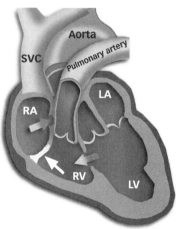

    ▶ Baun J: *Ob/Gyn Sonography: An Illustrated Review*. Pasadena, CA, Davies Publishing, 2016, p 181.

    ▶ Drose JA: *Fetal Echocardiography*, 2nd edition. St. Louis, Saunders Elsevier, 2010, pp 146–147.

139. A. Muscular atresia of the right atrial floor.

    Muscular atresia is the most common variation of the tricuspid valve, accounting for 76%–84% of cases. In this type, no tricuspid valvular tissue is found, and the floor of the right atrium is muscular.

    ▶ Drose JA: *Fetal Echocardiography*, 2nd edition. St. Louis, Saunders Elsevier, 2010, pp 146–147.

140. B. The relationship of the great arteries.

Tricuspid atresia is classified according to the relationship of the great arteries (GA). The three categories are subclassified according to the presence or absence of pulmonary stenosis/atresia or a ventricular septal defect (VSD). The three categories are:

- *Type I—Normal GA relationship: 69%*
  a. Pulmonary atresia without VSD
  b. Small (restrictive) VSD with pulmonary atresia
  c. Large (nonrestrictive) VSD without pulmonary stenosis

- *Type II—D-transposition of GA: 28%*
  a. Pulmonary atresia with VSD
  b. Pulmonary stenosis with VSD
  c. VSD with no pulmonary stenosis

- *Type III—L-transposition of GA: 3%*
  a. Subpulmonary stenosis with VSD
  b. Subaortic stenosis with VSD

▶ Drose JA: *Fetal Echocardiography*, 2nd edition. St. Louis, Saunders Elsevier, 2010, pp 146–147.

▶ Rosenthal A, Dick M: Tricuspid aresia. In Adams FH, Emmanouilides GC, Riemenschneider TA (eds): *Moss' Heart Disease in Infants, Children, and Adolescents*, 4th edition. Baltimore, Williams & Wilkins, 1989, p 903.

141. C. Anterior and to the left

In 69% of the cases of tricuspid atresia, the great arteries are normally related, i.e., the pulmonary artery is anterior and to the left of the aorta. See answer 140.

142. B. Ebstein anomaly.

The tricuspid valve leaflets must be evaluated thoroughly in order to diagnose Ebstein anomaly. It is the only defect in which the septal leaflet is displaced anteriorly.

▶ Drose JA: *Fetal Echocardiography*, 2nd edition. St. Louis, Saunders Elsevier, 2010, p 197.

143. A. Type I, normally related great arteries.

The relationship of the great arteries is normal in Type I in 69% of cases of tricuspid valve atresia. See the classification system in the answer to question 140.

▶ Drose JA: *Fetal Echocardiography*, 2nd edition. St. Louis, Saunders Elsevier, 2010, p 146.

144. C. Ebstein anomaly.

145. A. Anterior leaflet of tricuspid valve

The anterior leaflet of the tricuspid valve has a sail-like or stretched, redundant appearance because of the insufficiency of the tricuspid valve.

▶ Lundström N-R: Echocardiography in the diagnosis of Ebstein's anomaly of the tricuspid valve. Circulation 47:597–605, 1973.

146. E. Nearly 100%.

Situs inversus with extreme levocardia is quite rare. All cases will have an associated congenital heart defect, commonly corrected transposition of the great arteries, double-outlet right ventricle, and systemic venous anomalies.

▶ Drose JA: *Fetal Echocardiography*, 2nd edition. St. Louis, Saunders Elsevier, 2010, p 77.

147. D. 95%.

Situs solitus with dextrocardia is associated with a congenital heart defect in 95% of cases.

▶ Drose JA: *Fetal Echocardiography*, 2nd edition. St. Louis, Saunders Elsevier, 2010, p 76.

148. A. Less than 1%.

    Situs solitus is a normal body configuration that carries a risk for a congenital heart defect of less than 1% (8:1000).

    ▸ Drose JA: *Fetal Echocardiography*, 2nd edition. St. Louis, Saunders Elsevier, 2010, p 75.

149. D. Situs ambiguus.

150. E. A (pentalogy of Cantrell), B (limb–body wall complex), and C (amniotic band syndrome).

    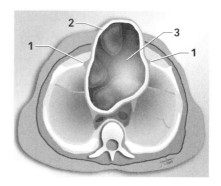

    In ectopia cordis, the heart is displaced from the chest cavity. Ectopia cordis is associated with pentalogy of Cantrell, limb–body wall complex, and amniotic band syndrome. The schematic represents an axial section demonstrating the heart herniated through a sternal defect. 1 = sternal defect, 2 = pericardium, 3 = herniated heart.

    ▸ Baun J: *Ob/Gyn Sonography: An Illustrated Review*. Pasadena, CA, Davies Publishing, 2016, p 186.

    ▸ Drose JA: *Fetal Echocardiography*, 2nd edition. St. Louis, Saunders Elsevier, 2010, pp 80–81.

151. A. Hypoplastic left heart syndrome.

    Extreme levocardia commonly occurs with conotruncal heart defects. Hypoplastic left heart syndrome is NOT a conotruncal defect. With hypoplastic left heart syndrome the heart position is usually normal.

152. E. Heterotaxy.

    Situs ambiguus (or situs ambiguous) and heterotaxy are synonymous. This is a type of cardiosplenic syndrome characterized by abnormalities of the vascular and visceral systems in which the usual left and right distribution of the thoracic and abdominal organs is disturbed.

    ▸ Drose JA: *Fetal Echocardiography*, 2nd edition. St. Louis, Saunders Elsevier, 2010, p 281.

153. E. All of the above.

    An abnormal heart position is often caused by an extracardiac malformation, congenital pulmonary airway malformation (CPAM, formerly called congenital cystic adenomatoid malformation or CCAM), congenital diaphragmatic hernia (CDH), bronchopulmonary sequestration, and pleural effusion.

    ▸ Drose JA: *Fetal Echocardiography*, 2nd edition. St. Louis, Saunders Elsevier, 2010, pp 80–86.

154. B. Ventricular septal defect.

    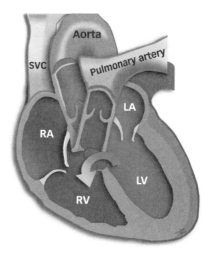

    A ventricular septal defect is an abnormal communication between the right and left ventricles that results
    in blood shunting from the left to the right ventricle (curved arrow). Ventricular septal defects account for approximately 30% of all congenital heart defects in live-borns (2–3 patients in 1000). Ventricular septal defects may be isolated or occur in association with other heart defects. SVC = superior vena cava, RA = right atrium, LA = left atrium, RV = right ventricle, LV = left ventricle. See also answer 159.

    ▸ Baun J: *Ob/Gyn Sonography: An Illustrated Review*. Pasadena, CA, Davies Publishing, 2016, p 173.

    ▸ Woodward PJ, Kennedy A, Sohaey R, et al: *Diagnostic Imaging: Obstetrics*. Salt Lake City, AMIRSYS, 2005, ch 6, p 21.

155. C. 6.7%.

An atrial septal defect is an abnormal communication between the right and left atria that results in abnormal shunting of blood (curved arrow) from the right atrium to the left atrium. SVC = superior vena cava, RA = right atrium, LA = left atrium, RV = right ventricle, LV = left ventricle.

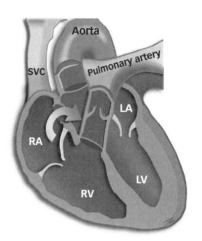

▶ Baun J: *Ob/Gyn Sonography: An Illustrated Review*. Pasadena, CA, Davies Publishing, 2016, p 175.

▶ Drose JA: *Fetal Echocardiography*, 2nd edition. St. Louis, Saunders Elsevier, 2010, p 92.

156. B. 3%–6%.

Aortic stenosis occurs in approximately 3%–6% of newborns with a congenital heart defect.

▶ Drose JA: *Fetal Echocardiography*, 2nd edition. St. Louis, Saunders Elsevier, 2010, p 169.

157. A. Excessive reabsorption of the septum primum.

▶ Drose JA: *Fetal Echocardiography*, 2nd edition. St. Louis, Saunders Elsevier, 2010, p 92.

158. B. Ventricular septal defect.

▶ Drose JA: *Fetal Echocardiography*, 2nd edition. St. Louis, Saunders Elsevier, 2010, p 105.

159. A. Ventricular septal defect.

Isolated ventricular septal defects (VSDs) are the most commonly recognized cardiac defect, accounting for approximately 30% of all cardiac defects recognized in live-borns and about 9.7% in fetuses. Bicuspid aortic valve is more common, but isolated VSDs are the most commonly recognized. See also answer 154.

▶ Drose JA: *Fetal Echocardiography*, 2nd edition. St. Louis, Saunders Elsevier, 2010, p 105.

▶ Ramaswamy P: Ventricular septal defects. Medscape, 2015. Available at http://emedicine.medscape.com/article/892980-overview.

160. A. Subaortic.

A subaortic ventricular septal defect is the most common type of ventricular septal defect in cases of tetralogy of Fallot.

161. B. Ostium secundum.

An ostium secundum atrial septal defect is the most common type of atrial septal defect, occurring in approximately 80% of cases. See also answer 155.

▶ Baun J: *Ob/Gyn Sonography: An Illustrated Review*. Pasadena, CA, Davies Publishing, 2016, p 175.

▶ Drose JA: *Fetal Echocardiography*, 2nd edition. St. Louis, Saunders Elsevier, 2010, p 94.

162. C. Ostium primum.

An ostium primum atrial septal defect is generally associated with the complex heart defect known as the atrioventricular septal defect.

▶ Drose JA: *Fetal Echocardiography*, 2nd edition. St. Louis, Saunders Elsevier, 2010, p 92.

163. A. Ventricular septal defect.

Ventricular septal defects (VSDs) are the most commonly recognized congenital cardiac defect, accounting for approximately 30%–50% of all diagnosed fetal heart lesions. After bicuspid aortic valve, VSDs are the most common (as well as most commonly recognized) heart defect.

▶ Drose JA: *Fetal Echocardiography*, 2nd edition. St. Louis, Saunders Elsevier, 2010, p 105.

▶ Ramaswamy P: Ventricular septal defects. Medscape, 2015. Available at http://emedicine.medscape.com/article/892980-overview.

164. B. Type B.

The most severe form of coarctation of the aorta is an interrupted aortic arch. Type B interruption is the most common. This interruption is between the left subclavian artery and the left common carotid artery. Refer to the diagram in answer 202.

165. A. Ventricular septal defect.

Ventricular septal defect (VSD) is present in nearly 100% of cases of double-outlet right ventricle (DORV). The type of DORV depends on where the VSD is. Pulmonary stenosis occurs in association with DORV in approximately 65%–70% of cases.

▶ Drose JA: *Fetal Echocardiography*, 2nd edition. St. Louis, Saunders Elsevier, 2010, pp 258, 263.

166. A. Subaortic.

Double-outlet right ventricle (DORV) is classified according to the location of the ventricular septal defect (VSD):

- *DORV with subaortic VSD (68%)—this is the most common*

- *DORV with subpulmonic VSD (Taussig-Bing type)*

- *DORV with doubly committed VSD (Fallot type)*

- *DORV with remote VSD*

167. E. Membranous.

The membranous ventricular septal defect (VSD) is the most common VSD, accounting for 75% of all VSDs. Almost all membranous VSDs are of the perimembranous type.

▶ Drose JA: *Fetal Echocardiography*, 2nd edition. St. Louis, Saunders Elsevier, 2010, pp 106–108.

168. A. Subaortic.

The anatomic locations of a ventricular septal defect in double-outlet left ventricle are the same as those for double-outlet right ventricle. The most common type is subaortic ventricular septal defect, observed in 48% of all cases.

169. E. All of the above.

170. C. Muscular ventricular septal defect. *(See Color Plate 1 on page xvii.)*

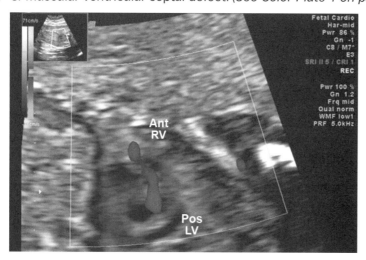

The image is a short-axis view of the ventricles. The muscular septum is demonstrated at this level. Blood flow is seen shunting across the septum. This is abnormal and is diagnosed as a muscular ventricular septal defect.

171. D. Differential diagnoses would include all of the above.

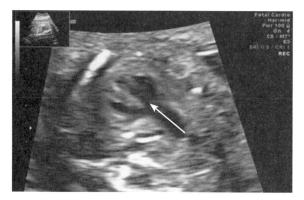

The image demonstrates an overriding aorta (arrow). The differential diagnoses must include tetralogy of Fallot, double-outlet right ventricle, and truncus arteriosus. Further imaging would be necessary to make the final diagnosis.

172. D. Coronary sinus atrial septal defect.

Coronary sinus atrial septal defects are rare, but when they occur they are often associated with a persistent left superior vena cava.

▸ Drose JA: *Fetal Echocardiography*, 2nd edition. St. Louis, Saunders Elsevier, 2010, p 91.

173. B. 1%–3%.

▸ Drose JA: *Fetal Echocardiography*, 2nd edition. St. Louis, Saunders Elsevier, 2010, p 163.

174. C. Pulmonic stenosis.

175. E. Both A (ostium primum atrial septal defect) and D (atrioventricular septal defect).

▸ Drose JA: *Fetal Echocardiography*, 2nd edition. St. Louis, Saunders Elsevier, 2010, p 11.

176. A. Extracellular matrix abnormality.

Extracellular matrix abnormalities affect the endocardial cushions of the heart. Atrioventricular septal defects are a result of the endocardial cushions failing to fuse. See also answer 97.

▸ Drose JA: *Fetal Echocardiography*, 2nd edition. St. Louis, Saunders Elsevier, 2010, pp 11–12, 119.

177. D. Atrioventricular septal defect.

The endocardial cushions develop from the extracellular matrix. They are involved in the formation of the semilunar (aortic and pulmonic) valves, atrioventricular (mitral and tricuspid) valves, and membranous septum. An atrioventricular septal defect (AVSD), also known as an atrioventricular canal, is a type of endocardial cushion defect resulting from incomplete closure of the embryonic endocardial cushions. This affects the atrial and ventricular septa and the tricuspid valve and/or mitral valve. A complete atrioventricular septal defect (seen in the schematic) consists of both atrial and ventricular septal defects with a common atrioventricular valve. It presents with a deformity secondary to narrowing of the left ventricular outflow tract. An incomplete atrioventricular septal defect consists of an atrial septal defect with separate mitral and tricuspid valve orifices. SVC = superior vena cava, RA = right atrium, LA = left atrium, RV = right ventricle, LV = left ventricle. See also answers 97 and 309.

▸ Baun J: *Ob/Gyn Sonography: An Illustrated Review.* Pasadena, CA, Davies Publishing, 2016, p 175.

▸ Drose JA: *Fetal Echocardiography*, 2nd edition. St. Louis, Saunders Elsevier, 2010, pp 11–12, 119.

▸ Moore KL, Persaud TVN: *The Developing Human*, 9th edition. Philadelphia, Saunders Elsevier, 2013, pp 299–300.

178. B. Tetralogy of Fallot.

Tetralogy of Fallot (TOF) accounts for 5%–10% (Woodward et al.) or 3.5%–7% (Drose) of all congenital heart defects. D-transposition of the great arteries is the next most frequent at 5.5%, and the others account for less than 3%. The schematic demonstrates the four main pathologic features of TOF: 1 = pulmonary artery stenosis, 2 = overriding aorta, 3 = right ventricular hypertrophy, 4 = ventricular septal defect. RV = right ventricle, LV = left ventricle, RA = right atrium, LA = left atrium, SVC = superior vena cava.

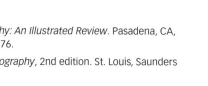

▶ Baun J: *Ob/Gyn Sonography: An Illustrated Review*. Pasadena, CA, Davies Publishing, 2016, p 176.

▶ Drose JA: *Fetal Echocardiography*, 2nd edition. St. Louis, Saunders Elsevier, 2010, pp 213–214.

▶ Woodward PJ, Kennedy A, Sohaey R, et al: *Diagnostic Imaging: Obstetrics*. Salt Lake City, AMIRSYS, 2005, ch 6, p 51.

179. C. Univentricular heart.

▶ Drose JA: *Fetal Echocardiography*, 2nd edition. St. Louis, Saunders Elsevier, 2010, p 162.

180. E. Tetralogy of Fallot.

181. A. Pulmonary atresia with an intact interventricular septum.

Pulmonary atresia with an intact ventricular septum is a defect caused by abnormal intracardiac blood flow. Blood flow is reduced, causing underdevelopment of the right ventricle. (Pulmonary atresia <u>with</u> *a ventricular septal defect would be considered a conontruncal heart defect.)*

▶ Drose JA: *Fetal Echocardiography*, 2nd edition. St. Louis, Saunders Elsevier, 2010, p 11.

182. C. Polysplenia.

183. A. Truncus arteriosus.

During organogenesis the truncus arteriosus—a single tubular embryonic conduit—arises cephalad from the bulbus cordis. Normally it will divide into the ascending aorta and the pulmonary trunk. When this partition fails, the condition is known as persistent truncus arteriosus. This leaves the heart with only one great artery coming off the two ventricles (see schematic), accompanied by a large ventricular septal defect and an abnormal truncal valve. 1 = truncus arteriosus, 2 = atrial septal defect, 3 = truncal valve, 4 = ventricular septal defect, RV = right ventricle, LV = left ventricle, RA = hypoplastic right atrium, LA = hypoplastic left atrium, SVC = superior vena cava, curved arrow = direction of blood flow. See also answer 190.

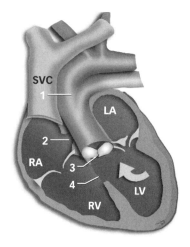

▶ Baun J: *Ob/Gyn Sonography: An Illustrated Review*. Pasadena, CA, Davies Publishing, 2016, p 179.

▶ Drose JA: *Fetal Echocardiography*, 2nd edition. St. Louis, Saunders Elsevier, 2010, p 223.

184. B. Left ventricle.

Truncus arteriosus can arise from the heart in various positions:

- *42% arise from the middle of the heart just superior to a ventricular septal defect.*

- *42% arise over the right ventricle.*

- *16% arise over the left ventricle.*

▶ Drose JA: *Fetal Echocardiography*, 2nd edition. St. Louis, Saunders Elsevier, 2010, pp 223–233.

185. C. Incomplete/partial.

    In the live-born, a partial atrioventricular septal defect is more common than the complete form.

    ▶ Woodward PJ, Kennedy A, Sohaey R, et al: *Diagnostic Imaging: Obstetrics*. Salt Lake City, AMIRSYS, 2005, ch 6, p 22.

186. C. Is connected to the right ventricle.

    Because of abnormal spiraling of the heart tube with d-transposition, the great arteries are malposed. The aorta is the anterior vessel and arises from the right ventricle, while the pulmonary artery is the posterior vessel and arises from the left ventricle.

187. D. Both A (the aorta is connected to the morphologic right ventricle) and C (the ventricles are inverted).

    In transposition of the great arteries, "dextro" (right) and "levo" (left) refer to the position of the aorta relative to the pulmonary artery. In both dextro- (d-) and levo- (l-) transposition, the aorta arises from the right ventricle while the pulmonary artery arises from the left ventricle. This is known as ventriculoarterial discordance. The major difference with l-transposition is that the ventricles are inverted. The morphologic right ventricle is on the left side of the heart and is the most posterior, while the morphologic left ventricle is on the right side and is anteriorly positioned. See also answer 190.

    ▶ Drose JA: *Fetal Echocardiography*, 2nd edition. St. Louis, Saunders Elsevier, 2010, pp 234, 239–240.
    ▶ Woodward PJ, Kennedy A, Sohaey R, et al: *Diagnostic Imaging: Obstetrics*. Salt Lake City, AMIRSYS, 2005, pp 54–57.

188. C. A rudimentary ventricular chamber.

    A rudimentary chamber is a nonfunctioning heart chamber. The chamber has no inlet and cannot receive flow from the atria and atrioventricular valve.

    ▶ Drose JA: *Fetal Echocardiography*, 2nd edition. St. Louis, Saunders Elsevier, 2010, pp 161–163.

189. B. 3 cusps.

    The single truncal valve has 3 cusps in 66% of cases. There may be as few as 2 or as many as 6 cusps.

    ▶ Drose JA: *Fetal Echocardiography*, 2nd edition. St. Louis, Saunders Elsevier, 2010, p 223.

190. D. The origin of the pulmonary arteries.

    Types I–IV (as classified by Collett and Edwards) are distinguished according to the origin of the pulmonary artery off the trunk in truncus arteriosus:

    - *Type I—Single short main pulmonary artery arises off the left lateral trunk (most common).*
    - *Type II—Two separate pulmonary arteries arise off the posterolateral trunk.*
    - *Type III—Widely spaced pulmonary arteries come off the lateral trunk.*
    - *Type IV—Pulmonary arteries come off the descending aorta.*

    See also answer 183.

    ▶ Collett RW, Edwards JE: Persistent truncus arteriosus: a classification according to anatomic types. Surg Clin North Am 29:1245–1270, 1949.
    ▶ Drose JA: *Fetal Echocardiography*, 2nd edition. St. Louis, Saunders Elsevier, 2010, pp 223–233.

191. B. Aorta.

192. D. Pulmonary artery.

    In both complete and corrected transposition, the aorta is connected to the morphologic right ventricle and the pulmonary artery is connected to the morphologic left ventricle:

    Complete TGA = RA − TV − RV − AO
    LA − MV − LV − PA
    Corrected TGA = RA − MV − LV − PA
    LA − TV − RV − AO

    Abbreviations: TGA = transposition of the great arteries, RA = right atrium, TV = tricuspid valve, RV = right ventricle, AO = aorta, LA = left atrium, MV = mitral valve, LV = left ventricle, PA = pulmonary artery.

193. E. Both C (short-axis view of the great vessels) and D (long-axis view of the great vessels).

In transposition of the great arteries (TGA) the four-chamber view appears normal. TGA presents with parallel great vessels arising from the outflow tracts. This is seen best in both the long-axis and short-axis views of the great vessels.

194. D. Tetralogy of Fallot.

Tetralogy of Fallot is the single most common malformation in children born with cyanotic heart disease.

▶ Kumar V, Abbas AK, Aster JC (eds): *Robbins Basic Pathology*, 9th edition. Philadelphia, Elsevier Saunders, 2013, pp 365–406.

195. D. Parallel.

Postnatally, the pulmonary and systemic circulations are parallel in complete transposition of the great arteries. The right ventricle serves as the systemic ventricle.

▶ Drose JA: *Fetal Echocardiography*, 2nd edition. St. Louis, Saunders Elsevier, 2010, pp 236–237.

196. B. Series.

Postnatally, the blood circulation in infants with corrected transposition is in series.

▶ Drose JA: *Fetal Echocardiography*, 2nd edition. St. Louis, Saunders Elsevier, 2010, p 239.

197. D. Atrioventricular septal defect.

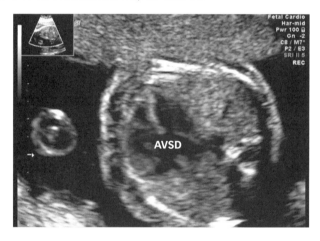

This large defect in the "crux" of the heart involves a large ventricular septal defect, ostium primum atrial septal defect, and single atrioventricular valve. This abnormal four-chamber view is characteristic of an atrioventricular septal defect.

198. C. Atrioventricular valves at the same level.

The atrioventricular valves appear to be at the same level, straight across in this image. This would be an abnormal finding, usually seen with atrioventricular septal defects. In the normal heart, the tricuspid valve is slightly offset from the mitral valve, being more apical in position than the mitral valve.

199. B. Tetralogy of Fallot.

Tetralogy of Fallot does NOT have parallel great vessels.

200. D. Pulmonary atresia.

Pulmonary atresia is characterized by abnormal blood flow and abnormal volume through the right side of the fetal heart.

201. C. Double-outlet right ventricle.

Double-outlet right ventricle (DORV) is embryologically a tissue-migration abnormality, whereas hypoplastic left heart syndrome (HLHS) is an abnormality of the intracardiac blood flow. HLHS is a progressive lesion primarily affecting the left side of the heart.

202. B. Type B.

CLASSIFICATION OF IAA

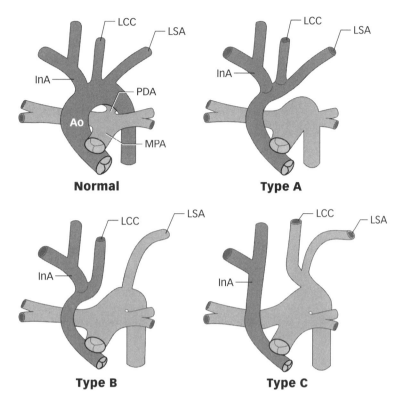

Normal

Type A

Type B

Type C

Source: Reprinted with permission from TheFetus.net.

Type B interruption of the aortic arch (IAA) is an interruption between the left common carotid (LCC) and left subclavian (LSA) arteries and is the most common. Type A occurs distal to the LSA, and Type C (least common) occurs between the innominate and LCC arteries.

Abbreviations: Ao = aorta, InA = innominate artery, LCC = left common carotid artery, LSA = left subclavian artery, MPA = main pulmonary artery, PDA = patent ductus arteriosus, RCC = right common carotid artery, RSA = right subclavian artery.

▶ Drose JA: *Fetal Echocardiography*, 2nd edition. St. Louis, Saunders Elsevier, 2010, pp 184–185.

203. A. Normally related great arteries.

The great arteries are normally related in the tetralogy of Fallot type of double-outlet right ventricle (DORV). This means the pulmonary artery is anterior and left of the aorta. The aorta overrides the septum to the right by 50% or more. Pulmonary stenosis is common in this form.

▶ Allan L, Hornberger L, Sharland G: *Textbook of Fetal Cardiology*. London, Greenwich Medical Media, 2000, p 274.

204. A. Coarctation of the aorta.

Incomplete development of left-heart structures (ventricle, atrium, mitral and aortic valves, and the aorta itself) result in hypoplastic left heart syndrome *or HLHS (see schematic)— the most common cause of postnatal congestive cardiac failure. HLHS is associated with coarctation of the aorta in approximately 70% of cases. SVC = superior vena cava, RA = right atrium, LA = left atrium, RV = right ventricle, LV = left ventricle.*

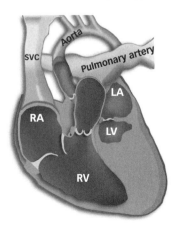

▶ Baun J: *Ob/Gyn Sonography: An Illustrated Review*. Pasadena, CA, Davies Publishing, 2016, p 181.

▶ Drose JA: *Fetal Echocardiography*, 2nd edition. St. Louis, Saunders Elsevier, 2010, p 142.

205. D. Between the left subclavian artery and the ductus arteriosus.

This is known as the isthmus.

206. D. Right ventricular hypertrophy.

Right ventricular hypertrophy may NOT *be apparent in utero because of the patent ductus arteriosus in the fetal circulation, which keeps the right ventricle at systemic pressure.*

207. D. Hypoplastic left heart syndrome.

Of all deaths related to cardiac disease in the pediatric population, 25% are related to hypoplastic left heart syndrome.

▸ Drose JA: *Fetal Echocardiography*, 2nd edition. St. Louis, Saunders Elsevier, 2010, p 133.

208. B. Hypoplastic left heart syndrome.

209. D. Bicuspid aortic valve.

Coarctation of the aorta is commonly associated with other heart malformations, most frequently bicuspid aortic valve. Bicuspid aortic valve occurs in approximately 85% of the cases of coarctation of the aorta. Other associations are aortic stenosis and ventricular septal defect.

▸ Drose JA: *Fetal Echocardiography*, 2nd edition. St. Louis, Saunders Elsevier, 2010, p 194.

210. C. Endocardial fibroelastosis.

Note that this diagnosis is suspected because of the clinical picture, but the final diagnosis is made by obtaining a pathologic specimen.

211. A. Aortic stenosis.

The four features that constitute the heart malformation known as tetralogy of Fallot are:

• *Perimembranous ventricular septal defect*

• *Overriding aorta*

• *Pulmonic stenosis*

• *Right ventricular hypertrophy (which may not be seen in utero)*

▸ Drose JA: *Fetal Echocardiography*, 2nd edition. St. Louis, Saunders Elsevier, 2010, pp 211–212.

212. C. Hypoplastic left heart syndrome.

Hypoplastic left heart syndrome *consists of several lesions that obstruct the left heart and occur in varying degrees: aortic atresia, hypoplastic aorta, hypoplastic or atretic mitral valve, and small left atrium and ventricle.*

▸ Drose JA: *Fetal Echocardiography*, 2nd edition. St. Louis, Saunders Elsevier, 2010, p 131.

213. D. A (cor triatriatum), B (parachute mitral valve), and C (supravalvular mitral ring).

214. B. Right ventricular diameter greater than left ventricular diameter.

Coarctation of the aorta may be difficult to diagnose in utero. An indirect sign of narrowing of the aorta is right-ventricle-to-left-ventricle disproportion, with the right ventricle larger than the left ventricle. This disproportion is caused by decreased flow through the aorta as a result of the narrowing and elevated left atrial pressure. This results in blood shunting left to right across the foramen ovale back into the right atrium and across the tricuspid valve, filling the right ventricle. This increased blood flow causes increased volume in the right ventricle, thereby increasing right ventricular diameter.

215. D. Both A (endocardial fibroelastosis) and B (hypoplastic left heart).

The very small left ventricle with thickened, echogenic, calcified walls is a result of the sequence involved in hypoplastic left heart syndrome with endocardial fibroelastosis. Endocardial fibroelastosis results when blood flow exiting the left heart is restricted due to the narrowed aorta. The blood remains stagnant in the left ventricle, producing fibrin that adheres to the walls of the left ventricle. The left ventricular walls become thick and echogenic. The left ventricle is unable to contract and has poor function.

216. C. Double-inlet single ventricle, left ventricle morphology.

The most common form of univentricular heart is double-inlet single ventricle, left ventricle morphology, with a left-sided rudimentary right ventricle chamber (L-loop). Using Hallermann's modification of Van Praagh's univentricular heart classification, this is Type A with L-loop. Each anatomic type of univentricular heart can develop from either a levo or a dextro bulboventricular loop (L-loop or D-loop), and the anatomy of each type is different. The basic Van Praagh types are:

Type	Principal Malformation
A	*Absent right ventricular sinus (with D-loop or L-loop)*
B	*Absent left ventricular sinus (with D-loop or L-loop)*
C	*Absent or rudimentary ventricular septum (with D-loop or L-loop)*
D	*Absent right and left ventricular sinuses and absent ventricular septum (with D-loop or L-loop)*

Furthermore, these lesions are subclassified by the positions of the great vessels—whether (1) normal, (2) with aorta anterior and to the right, or (3) with aorta anterior and to the left. Type A, subtype 3, accounts for approximately 60% of cases.

▸ Drose JA: *Fetal Echocardiography*, 2nd edition. St. Louis, Saunders Elsevier, 2010, pp 160–161.

▸ Hallermann FJ, Davis GD, Ritter DG, et al: Roentgenographic features of common ventricle. Radiology 87:409–423, 1966.

217. B. Double-outlet left ventricle.

When both the aorta and the pulmonary artery arise from the left ventricle, the defect is termed double-outlet left ventricle.

218. A. Univentricular heart.

Univentricular heart is the diagnosis. Tetralogy of Fallot would show two normal sized ventricular chambers with a malalignment type VSD. Ebstein anomaly would present with a dilated right atrium and abnormal septal leaflet. Pericardial effusion is not present. The heart does not appear normal, because the left ventricle is larger than the right. Therefore univentricular heart is the best answer.

219. C. Type C.

Type C is the most lethal. See answer 216.

▸ Drose JA: *Fetal Echocardiography*, 2nd edition. St. Louis, Saunders Elsevier, 2010, p 165.

220. B. Type B interruption.

Type B interruptions occur at the level of the left common carotid artery and the left subclavian artery. See answer 202.

221. C. Type C interruption.

The least common type of interrupted aortic arch occurs between the innominate (brachiocephalic) and the left common carotid arteries. This is termed Type C *interruption. See answer 202.*

▸ Drose JA: *Fetal Echocardiography*, 2nd edition. St. Louis, Saunders Elsevier, 2010, pp 184–185.

222. C. Right-to-left shunting at the atrial level.

Right-to-left shunting at the atrial level would NOT *occur because there is an obligate left-to-right shunt at the atrial level as a result of there being no egress for blood in the left atrium. There would still be right-to-left shunting at the ductal level, however.*

223. D. Both A (an atrial septal defect) and C (a right-to-left shunt at the atrial level).

▸ Drose JA: *Fetal Echocardiography*, 2nd edition. St. Louis, Saunders Elsevier, 2010, p 245.

224. A. Supracardiac.

The supracardiac type of total anomalous pulmonary venous return (TAPVR) occurs most frequently, accounting for approximately 44% of cases.

▶ Drose JA: *Fetal Echocardiography*, 2nd edition. St. Louis, Saunders Elsevier, 2010, p 245.

225. B. Scimitar syndrome.

Anomalous venous drainage of the right lower and middle lobes occurring in association with right lung hypoplasia is termed the scimitar syndrome. *One or more of the pulmonary veins drain anomalously into the inferior vena cava, and abnormal arterial flow goes into the right lung.*

▶ Allan L, Hornberger L, Sharland G: *Textbook of Fetal Cardiology*. London, Greenwich Medical Media, 2000, p 106.

226. B. Sinus venosus atrial septal defect.

▶ Drose JA: *Fetal Echocardiography*, 2nd edition. St. Louis, Saunders Elsevier, 2010, p 91.

227. D. Both A (enlarged right ventricle) and B (prominent pulmonary artery).

Diagnosis of total anomalous pulmonary venous return (TAPVR) in the fetus is very difficult. The right ventricle and pulmonary artery will be enlarged due to increased blood flow into the right heart. The pulmonary veins drain directly or indirectly into the right atrium instead of the left atrium. When enlargement of the right ventricle and pulmonary artery is present, investigation of the pulmonary veins must be performed to rule out anomalous pulmonary venous connections.

▶ Drose JA: *Fetal Echocardiography*, 2nd edition. St. Louis, Saunders Elsevier, 2010, pp 250–252.

228. C. Infracardiac.

In almost all cases of infracardiac total anomalous pulmonary venous return (TAPVR) there is some type of obstruction of the venous return to the heart. The obstruction can occur at any level.

▶ Drose JA: *Fetal Echocardiography*, 2nd edition. St. Louis, Saunders Elsevier, 2010, p 247.

229. A. Supracardiac.

Supracardiac total anomalous pulmonary venous return (TAPVR) is rarely associated with venous obstruction.

▶ Drose JA: *Fetal Echocardiography*, 2nd edition. St. Louis, Saunders Elsevier, 2010, p 247.

230. A. Atrial septal defect.

With total anomalous pulmonary venous return (TAPVR) there is almost always a right-to-left shunt—atrial septal defect—allowing blood to return to the left heart and systemic circulation.

▶ Drose JA: *Fetal Echocardiography*, 2nd edition. St. Louis, Saunders Elsevier, 2010, pp 253–254.

231. C. Sinus venosus atrial septal defect.

80%–90% of sinus venosus defects of the superior vena cava type are associated with an anomalous pulmonary connection of the right superior pulmonary vein to the right atrium or superior vena cava.

▶ Drose JA: *Fetal Echocardiography*, 2nd edition. St. Louis, Saunders Elsevier, 2010, pp 91, 101.

232. A. Ebstein anomaly.

233. B. Absent pulmonic valve syndrome.

234. D. Pulmonary atresia with an intact interventricular septum.

▶ Drose JA: *Fetal Echocardiography*, 2nd edition. St. Louis, Saunders Elsevier, 2010, p 145.

235. A. Pulmonary stenosis.

Pulmonary stenosis occurs in 65%–70% of the cases of double-outlet right ventricle.

▶ Drose JA: *Fetal Echocardiography*, 2nd edition. St. Louis, Saunders Elsevier, 2010, p 263.

236. D. A (severe tricuspid regurgitation) and C (Ebstein anomaly).

Bowing of the ventricular septum toward the left ventricle is due to volume load in the right ventricle.

237. B. Agenesis of the ductus arteriosus.

Agenesis of the ductus arteriosus occurs in 50%–75% of cases of truncus arteriosus. A right-sided aortic arch is present in 15%–30% of patients. Interruption of the aortic arch has also been associated with truncus arteriosus.

▶ Drose JA: *Fetal Echocardiography*, 2nd edition. St. Louis, Saunders Elsevier, 2010, p 223.

238. C. Side by side.

There are four types of double-outlet right ventricle (DORV) based on the relationship of the great arteries:

1. Aorta right and posterior to pulmonary artery (PA)—normal

2. Aorta right and lateral to PA—"side by side" (most common)

3. Aorta left and anterior to PA—levomalposition

4. Aorta anterior to PA—dextromalposition (common)

▶ Drose JA: *Fetal Echocardiography*, 2nd edition. St. Louis, Saunders Elsevier, 2010, pp 256–257.

239. E. All of the above.

Right-sided aortic arch is commonly associated with conotruncal heart defects:
- *Truncus arteriosus = 50%*
- *Tetralogy of Fallot = 25%*
- *Complete transposition of the great arteries (TGA) = 20%*
- *Pulmonary atresia = 5%*

▶ Drose JA: *Fetal Echocardiography*, 2nd edition. St. Louis, Saunders Elsevier, 2010, p 11.

240. E. All of the above.

If you see a ventricular septal defect (VSD) with aortic override, the differential diagnoses are double-outlet right ventricle, truncus arteriosus, tetralogy of Fallot, and pulmonary atresia with VSD. See the image in answer 171.

241. A. Double-outlet right ventricle with a subaortic ventricular septal defect.

Double-outlet right ventricle with a subaortic ventricular septal defect is the most common, occurring in 68% of cases.

242. B. Subpulmonic ventricular septal defect with side-by-side great vessels.

The classic Taussig-Bing physiology is like that in transposition of the great arteries postnatally.

▶ Drose JA: *Fetal Echocardiography*, 2nd edition. St. Louis, Saunders Elsevier, 2010, pp 256–259.

243. D. Pulmonic stenosis.

▶ Drose JA: *Fetal Echocardiography*, 2nd edition. St. Louis, Saunders Elsevier, 2010, p 263.

244. A. Ebstein anomaly (dysplastic tricuspid valve).

This image is characteristic of Ebstein anomaly because of the massive dilatation of the right atrium. The right atrium fills the entire fetal chest. The right ventricle is also enlarged compared to the left.

245. E. Pulmonic stenosis.

Ebstein anomaly is highly associated with pulmonary stenosis because of the atrialization of the right ventricle.

246. C. Lithium.

Ebstein anomaly has been associated with maternal ingestion of lithium carbonate, a drug used in the treatment of bipolar disorder.

▶ Drose JA: *Fetal Echocardiography*, 2nd edition. St. Louis, Saunders Elsevier, 2010, p 198.

247. A. Secundum atrial septal defect.

248. D. Tissue-migration abnormality.

The defect appears to involve the conotruncus and the conotruncal septum. These defects fall into the category of a tissue-migration abnormality. The atrial septum at the level of the septum secundum can NOT be evaluated from these images.

249. A. Double-outlet right ventricle.

In double-outlet right ventricle (DORV), both the aorta and the pulmonary artery arise from the right ventricle. More than 50% of the aorta must override the septum to the right ventricle to diagnose DORV. This is known as the "50% rule": 50% to the right indicates DORV, 50% to the left indicates tetralogy of Fallot. SVC = superior vena cava, RA = right atrium, LA = left atrium, RV = right ventricle, LV = left ventricle. See also answer 238.

250. B. Dilated pulmonary arteries.

This image is taken at the level of the trifurcation of the pulmonary artery. The pulmonary trunk and the branch pulmonary arteries are massively dilated.

251. C. Absent pulmonic valve syndrome.

Absence of the pulmonic valve causes massive distention of the pulmonary artery and its branches.

252. B. Interrupted inferior vena cava with azygos vein continuation.

In the normal four-chamber view, only the aorta should be seen posterior to the heart. If two vessels are visualized, the most common anatomic explanation is an interrupted IVC with an azygos vein that continues to the heart.

▶ Drose JA: *Fetal Echocardiography*, 2nd edition. St. Louis, Saunders Elsevier, 2010, pp 281–288.

253. D. Polysplenia.

An interrupted inferior vena cava with an azygos vein continuation is the anatomic anomaly most commonly associated with polysplenia.

▶ Drose JA: *Fetal Echocardiography*, 2nd edition. St. Louis, Saunders Elsevier, 2010, p 283.

254. C. Anomalous pulmonary venous connections.

Of those fetuses with sinus venosus atrial septal defects, 80%–90% will have an anomalous pulmonary venous connection to the right atrium or the superior vena cava.

▶ Drose JA: *Fetal Echocardiography*, 2nd edition. St. Louis, Saunders Elsevier, 2010, p 101.

255. E. Agenesis of the ductus venosus.

With agenesis of the ductus venosus, blood entering the fetus through the umbilical vein flows into the inferior vena cava (IVC) and is abruptly terminated because of the absent ductus venosus. This rare (1:2500) condition causes dilatation of the IVC due to extrahepatic sources of umbilical vein blood flow such as the femoral vein, iliac vein, and inferior vena cava. Although one might argue for choice C, "Anomalous pulmonary venous connections"—which, when infracardiac, can cause IVC dilatation—in utero only 10% of blood flow goes to the lungs and there is not much blood flow in the pulmonary veins to dilate the IVC in total anomalous pulmonary venous return (TAPVR), so anomalous pulmonary venous connection is NOT correct.

256. E. Right atrium.

A coronary sinus atrial septal defect (ASD) will be found at the ostium of the coronary sinus in the right atrium. In this defect the coronary sinus is dilated as a result of the increased flow in this area.

▶ Drose JA: *Fetal Echocardiography*, 2nd edition. St. Louis, Saunders Elsevier, 2010, p 91.

257. A. Left superior vena cava.

Coronary sinus atrial septal defects are rare, but a common association with this defect is a left superior vena cava, which enters the upper left aspect of the left atrium.

▸ Drose JA: *Fetal Echocardiography*, 2nd edition. St. Louis, Saunders Elsevier, 2010, p 91.

258. E. Persistent left superior vena cava.

259. B. Persistent left superior vena cava.

A persistent left superior vena cava enters the left atrium and is characterized as a cyst-like structure along the wall of the left atrium. The left superior vena cava then travels posteriorly and enters into the coronary sinus.

260. C. Persistent left superior vena cava.

Once the persistent left superior vena cava enters the left atrium it travels posteriorly and enters into the coronary sinus. The coronary sinus becomes dilated as a result of the increased blood flow.

261. D. Dilated coronary sinus.

262. B. Persistent left superior vena cava.

The persistent left superior vena cava is seen as a cyst-like structure along the wall of the left atrium. The left superior vena cava enters into the left atrium and travels posteriorly into the coronary sinus.

263. C. Persistent right umbilical vein.

The intra-abdominal umbilical vein should be seen coursing away from the stomach bubble toward the fetal liver. This is visualized at the level of the fetal stomach in the transverse scan plane.

264. E. Both C (left atrial isomerism) and D (polysplenia syndrome).

Left atrial isomerism *and* polysplenia syndrome *are synonymous. In 65%–70% of polysplenia syndrome cases there is an absent intrahepatic inferior vena cava with collateral drainage via the azygos vein.*

▸ Drose JA: *Fetal Echocardiography*, 2nd edition. St. Louis, Saunders Elsevier, 2010, pp 281–282.

265. A. Rhabdomyoma.

Rhabdomyoma—the most common cardiac tumor of infants and children—occurs in 60% of cardiac tumor cases. Rhabdomyoma is also the most common cardiac tumor in fetuses, although the incidence of all fetal cardiac tumors is only 0.14%.

▸ Drose JA: *Fetal Echocardiography*, 2nd edition. St. Louis, Saunders Elsevier, 2010, p 268.

266. E. Tuberous sclerosis.

▸ Drose JA: *Fetal Echocardiography*, 2nd edition. St. Louis, Saunders Elsevier, 2010, p 272.

267. C. Intrapericardial teratoma.

Intrapericardial teratomas are unique because of their large size and encapsulation. They are usually found attached to the base of the heart by a stalk.

268. C. Myxoma.

Myxomas are generally NOT *seen in utero, but they are the most common primary cardiac tumor in the adult.*

▸ Drose JA: *Fetal Echocardiography*, 2nd edition. St. Louis, Saunders Elsevier, 2010, p 269.

269. A. Echogenic foci.

270. E. Both B (left atrial isomerism) and C (bilateral left-sidedness).

Polysplenia is characterized by bilateral left-sidedness or left atrial isomerism. It is termed polysplenia *because of the abnormal multiple ("poly") spleens.*

▶ Drose JA: *Fetal Echocardiography*, 2nd edition. St. Louis, Saunders Elsevier, 2010, pp 281–282.

271. B. Holt-Oram syndrome (heart-hand syndrome).

▶ Drose JA: *Fetal Echocardiography*, 2nd edition. St. Louis, Saunders Elsevier, 2010, p 94.

272. B. Polysplenia syndrome.

▶ Drose JA: *Fetal Echocardiography*, 2nd edition. St. Louis, Saunders Elsevier, 2010, pp 281–282.

273. D. All of the above.

274. E. All of the above.

▶ Drose JA: *Fetal Echocardiography*, 2nd edition. St. Louis, Saunders Elsevier, 2010, pp 142, 174, 192.

275. C. Noonan syndrome.

276. B. Polysplenia syndrome.

▶ Drose JA: *Fetal Echocardiography*, 2nd edition. St. Louis, Saunders Elsevier, 2010, p 282.

277. A. Down syndrome (trisomy 21).

Down syndrome is associated with 40% to 50% of all cases of atrioventricular septal defect (AVSD). When an AVSD is associated with tetralogy of Fallot, the most common associated condition is Down syndrome.

278. E. Asplenia syndrome.

279. E. A (asplenia syndrome) and D (right atrial isomerism).

Asplenia syndrome *and* right atrial isomerism *are synonymous terms. The position of the inferior vena cava (IVC) in the fetal thorax is altered as a result of the abnormal organ arrangements. In contrast,* polysplenia syndrome *has an interrupted IVC with an azygos vein that continues to the heart and is seen at the level of the four-chamber heart view.*

280. C. Turner syndrome.

Turner syndrome is related to approximately 45% of all cases of coarctation of the aorta.

▶ Allan L, Hornberger L, Sharland G: *Textbook of Fetal Cardiology*. London, Greenwich Medical Media, 2000, p 31.

281. A. Down syndrome (trisomy 21).

Down syndrome (trisomy 21) is associated with approximately 40% of cases of atrioventricular septal defect.

▶ Allan L, Hornberger L, Sharland G: *Textbook of Fetal Cardiology*. London, Greenwich Medical Media, 2000, p 6.

282. E. All of the above.

Univentricular heart commonly occurs with various heart defects, syndromes, and chromosomal abnormalities. Heterotaxy and Edwards syndromes are the most commonly associated syndromes. Coarctation of the aorta and interrupted aortic arch are the most commonly associated cardiac defects, along with valvular stenoses and atresias. See also answer 216.

▶ Drose JA: *Fetal Echocardiography*, 2nd edition. St. Louis, Saunders Elsevier, 2010, pp 166–167.

283. D. DiGeorge syndrome.

Cases of Type B interruption with a ventricular septal defect will be associated with DiGeorge syndrome (22q11.2 deletion syndrome) 50% or more of the time.

284. C. Williams syndrome.

     Supravalvular aortic stenosis occurs commonly in Williams syndrome.

     ▸ Drose JA: *Fetal Echocardiography*, 2nd edition. St. Louis, Saunders Elsevier, 2010, p 170.

285. B. Noonan syndrome.

     Pulmonic valve stenosis caused by a dysplastic pulmonic valve is a common finding in patients with Noonan syndrome.

     ▸ Drose JA: *Fetal Echocardiography*, 2nd edition. St. Louis, Saunders Elsevier, 2010, p 179.

286. D. DiGeorge syndrome.

     Truncus arteriosus is associated with multiple syndromes, DiGeorge syndrome (22q11.2 deletion syndrome) being the most common. Truncus arteriosus has been reported in 33% of patients with DiGeorge syndrome.

     ▸ Drose JA: *Fetal Echocardiography*, 2nd edition. St. Louis, Saunders Elsevier, 2010, p 231.

287. B. Asplenia syndrome.

     Cardiac defects are often associated with asplenia syndrome. The incidence of an atrioventricular septal defect is 85%, and double-outlet right ventricle has an incidence of 80%.

     ▸ Drose JA: *Fetal Echocardiography*, 2nd edition. St. Louis, Saunders Elsevier, 2010, p 282.

288. D. Cor triatriatum.

     Shone syndrome—also known as Shone complex—is a series of four obstructive or potentially obstructive left-sided cardiac lesions:

     - *Supravalvular mitral ring*

     - *Parachute deformity of the mitral valve*

     - *Subaortic stenosis*

     - *Coarctation of the aorta*

     It may be complete (all four lesions) or incomplete (with fewer than four lesions).

289. E. All of the above.

     Asplenia is characterized by bilateral right-sidedness or right atrial isomerism. The fetus will have an absent spleen. Swedish pediatrician and pathologist Biörn Ivemark first described asplenia in 1955—hence asplenia is also known as Ivemark syndrome.

     ▸ Drose JA: *Fetal Echocardiography*, 2nd edition. St. Louis, Saunders Elsevier, 2010, p 281.

290. C. Polysplenia syndrome.

     Among atrioventricular septal defect cases, 15%–20% are associated with heterotaxy syndrome, specifically left atrial isomerism (also known as polysplenia syndrome).

     ▸ Woodward PJ, Kennedy A, Sohaey R, et al: *Diagnostic Imaging: Obstetrics*. Salt Lake City, AMIRSYS, 2005, ch 6, p 23.

291. B. Right atrial isomerism.

     Right atrial isomerism is also known as asplenia syndrome. Asplenia is commonly associated with cardiac defects. Atrioventricular septal defects have been associated with 85%–95% of cases. Right heart obstruction is also common, including pulmonary atresia or pulmonary stenosis and double-outlet right ventricle, both with an 80% occurrence.

     ▸ Drose JA: *Fetal Echocardiography*, 2nd edition. St. Louis, Saunders Elsevier, 2010, p 281.

292. A. Polysplenia syndrome.

In 65%–70% of polysplenia syndrome cases there is an absent intrahepatic inferior vena cava with collateral drainage via the azygos vein. Other cardiac anomalies occur frequently with polysplenia, including left-sided heart obstruction.

▸ Drose JA: *Fetal Echocardiography*, 2nd edition. St. Louis, Saunders Elsevier, 2010, pp 281–282.

293. C. Pulmonic valve stenosis.

Pulmonic valve stenosis caused by a dysplastic pulmonic valve is frequently found in patients with Noonan syndrome.

▸ Drose JA: *Fetal Echocardiography*, 2nd edition. St. Louis, Saunders Elsevier, 2010, pp 174–175.

294. D. Turner syndrome.

In about 75% of fetuses with cystic hygroma, there is a chromosomal abnormality, and in 95% of these cases the abnormality is Turner syndrome. See also answer 319.

▸ Nicolaides KD, Sebire NJ, Snijder RJM: *The 11–14 Week Scan: The Diagnosis of Fetal Abnormalities*. London, Parthenon, 1999,
pp 14–15.

PART 3
Patient Care

295. E. All of the above.

296. E. Either A (washing hands thoroughly with soap and water for 40–60 seconds after every examination) or B (rubbing hands with an alcohol-based product for 20–30 seconds until dry after every examination) is acceptable.

    Hand washing and hand rubbing are major components of the Standard Precautions (also known as the Universal Precautions) and one of the most effective methods to prevent transmission of pathogens associated with health care. According to the Standard Precautions: "Hand hygiene procedures include the use of alcohol-based hand rubs (containing 60–95% alcohol) and handwashing with soap and water. Alcohol-based hand rub is the preferred method for decontaminating hands, except when hands are visibly soiled (e.g., dirt, blood, body fluids), or after caring for patients with known or suspected infectious diarrhea (e.g., Clostridium difficile, norovirus), in which case soap and water should be used. Hand hygiene stations should be strategically placed to ensure easy access."

    ▶ Centers for Disease Control and Prevention: Standard Precautions: hand hygiene. Available at http://www.cdc.gov/HAI/settings/outpatient/basic-infection-control-prevention-plan-2011/standard-precautions.html.

297. E. Both C (perform the examination wearing protective gloves) and D (clean the transducer after the procedure with a recommended equipment disinfectant).

    The sonographer must wear gloves to prevent contact with the rash and spreading the rash. Also, it is mandatory that proper cleaning and disinfecting of the ultrasound equipment are performed before use for another patient.

298. D. All of the above.

    All these precautions should be taken. The probe needs to be both wiped clean and sanitized.

299. E. All of the above.

    In addition to blood, the Occupational Safety and Health Administration defines "other potentially infectious materials" (OPIM) to include the following human bodily fluids: semen, vaginal secretions, cerebrospinal fluid, synovial fluid, pleural fluid, pericardial fluid, peritoneal fluid, amniotic fluid, saliva in dental procedures, any body fluid that is visibly contaminated with blood, and all body fluids in situations where it is difficult or impossible to differentiate between body fluids.

    ▶ Occupational Safety and Health Administration: Healthcare wide hazards: (Lack of) Universal Precautions. Available at https://www.osha.gov/SLTC/etools/hospital/hazards/univprec/univ.html.

300. C. Wearing protective clothing and eyewear.

    Wear gloves, clean equipment, discard used linen, and always maintain proper hand hygiene (through hand washing or rubbing) with every patient. Fetal echocardiography does NOT require the use of protective clothing or eyewear, because the risk of contacting body fluids, including blood, is very low.

301. B. Occupational Safety and Health Administration (OSHA).

    The Standard Precautions (formerly Universal Precautions) were developed by OSHA as an "approach to infection control to treat all human blood and certain human body fluids as if they were known to be infectious for HIV, HBV and other blood-borne pathogens." Some of these practices include using gloves, masks, and gowns if exposure to blood or "other potentially infectious materials" (OPIM) is anticipated, as well as using engineering and work practice controls to limit such exposure.

    ▶ Occupational Safety and Health Administration: Standard precautions: protecting yourself from risk. Available at http://www.swcec.org/modules/groups/homepagefiles/cms/2286232/File/OSHA%20and%20Standard%20Precuations%20%202012.pdf.

PART 4

Integration of Data

302. D. Echogenic foci.

     Echogenic foci constitute an incidental finding and may be seen in approximately 3%–4% of all second trimester fetuses. In a low-risk patient, an echogenic focus is considered normal.

     ▶ Drose JA: *Fetal Echocardiography*, 2nd edition. St. Louis, Saunders Elsevier, 2010, pp 60–61.

     ▶ Woodward PJ, Kennedy A, Sohaey R, et al: *Diagnostic Imaging: Obstetrics*. Salt Lake City, AMIRSYS, 2005, ch 6, p 6.

303. D. 8 in 1000 infants.

304. C. Ventricular septal defect.

     About 60% of ventricular septal defects occur in isolation, accounting for approximately 30% of all cardiac defects in live-born infants. After bicuspid aortic valves, ventricular septal defects are the most commonly recognized heart lesion.

     ▶ Drose JA: *Fetal Echocardiography*, 2nd edition. St. Louis, Saunders Elsevier, 2010, p 105.

     ▶ Ramaswamy P: Ventricular septal defects. Medscape, 2015. Available at http://emedicine.medscape.com/article /892980-overview.

305. C. 6.5%.

     Type II diabetes mellitus is diagnosed when the level of hemoglobin A1C is 6.5% or higher on two separate occasions.

306. D. Rhabdomyoma.

     Rhabdomyomas are the most common cardiac tumor in fetuses. There is a high association with tuberous sclerosis. Rhabdomyomas may be multiple. They are usually located in the ventricles or septum.

307. C. 13%.

     The incidence of an abnormal karyotype in live-born infants with a congenital heart defect is approximately 13%. The incidence of an abnormal karyotype in fetuses with a congenital heart defect has been reported to be approximately 35%.

     ▶ Drose JA: *Fetal Echocardiography*, 2nd edition. St. Louis, Saunders Elsevier, 2010, p 19.

308. C. 50%.

     An abnormal karyotype carries an increased risk for a heart defect. Trisomy 21 carries a risk of approximately 40%–50%.

     ▶ Drose JA: *Fetal Echocardiography*, 2nd edition. St. Louis, Saunders Elsevier, 2010, p 19.

309. A. Trisomy 21 (Down syndrome).

     Atrioventricular septal defects have been associated with multiple syndromes and chromosomal abnormalities. In patients with trisomy 21, atrioventricular septal defects account for 40% of heart defects. See also answers 97 and 177.

     ▶ Drose JA: *Fetal Echocardiography*, 2nd edition.St. Louis, Saunders Elsevier, 2010, p 122.

310. E. Both B (trisomy 13 [Patau syndrome]) and D (trisomy 18 [Edwards syndrome]).

     The association of both trisomy13 (Patau syndrome) and trisomy 18 (Edwards syndrome) with a heart defect is nearly 100%.

     ▶ Drose JA: *Fetal Echocardiography*, 2nd edition. St. Louis, Saunders Elsevier, 2010, p 19.

311. A. DiGeorge syndrome.

     DiGeorge syndrome is also known as 22q11.2 deletion syndrome.

312. E. All of the above.

     All the syndromes listed are known to be associated with congenital heart disease.

313. C. 10%.

     With two or more siblings affected with a heart defect, the risk to the fetus is 10%.

     ▶ Drose JA: *Fetal Echocardiography*, 2nd edition. St. Louis, Saunders Elsevier, 2010, p 17.

314. C. 10%–12%.

     If the mother of a fetus is affected, the risk to the fetus is 10%–12%.

     ▶ Drose JA: *Fetal Echocardiography*, 2nd edition. St. Louis, Saunders Elsevier, 2010, p 17.

315. B. 2%–4%.

     When a single sibling is affected, the risk to the fetus is 2%–4%.

     ▶ Drose JA: *Fetal Echocardiography*, 2nd edition. St. Louis, Saunders Elsevier, 2010, p 17.

316. A. Ventricular septal defect.

317. A. Oligohydramnios.

318. E. A (it suggests the presence of structural heart defects) and D (it may indicate fetal cardiac dysrhythmias).

     Nonimmune hydrops fetalis can result from both structural heart defects and dysrhythmias and is therefore an indication for fetal echocardiography. Immune hydrops is associated with Rh isoimmunization and alloimmune hemolytic disease.

     ▶ Baun J: *Ob/Gyn Sonography: An Illustrated Review*. Pasadena, CA, Davies Publishing, 2016, pp 302–303.

     ▶ Drose JA: *Fetal Echocardiography*, 2nd edition. St. Louis, Saunders Elsevier, 2010, p 26.

319. B. 2.5 mm.

     Nuchal translucency (NT) refers to the collection of lymphatic fluid found in the posterior neck region of the embryo, which is normal in early pregnancy but can indicate genetic anomalies if it exceeds normal values. From menstrual weeks 11 to 14, the normal nuchal translucency is 1.0 to 2.5 mm as measured by ultrasound. NT measurements that exceed this finding are associated with a risk of congenital heart disease that increases as NT thickness increases. See also answers 294, 352, 353, and 354.

     ▶ Baun J: *Ob/Gyn Sonography: An Illustrated Review*. Pasadena, CA, Davies Publishing, 2016, pp 13, 276–277.

     ▶ Drose JA: *Fetal Echocardiography*, 2nd edition.St. Louis, Saunders Elsevier, 2010, pp 26–27.

     ▶ Guraya SS: The associations of nuchal translucency and fetal abnormalities: significance and implications. J Clin Diagn Res 7:936–941, 2013.

320. C. Atrial flutter.

     Atrial flutter is a tachyarrhythmia with an atrial rate between 300 and 500 beats per minute (bpm). The ventricular response is variable.

     ▶ Drose JA: *Fetal Echocardiography*, 2nd edition. St. Louis, Saunders Elsevier, 2010, p 308.

321. B. Gastroschisis.

Some extracardiac anomalies carry a 25%–45% risk for an associated complex heart defect, while other fetal defects do NOT carry any increased risk for a heart defect. Gastroschisis, unlike an omphalocele, is usually an isolated defect. It would NOT warrant any further fetal echocardiographic exam. Extracardiac anomalies associated with an increased risk of developmental heart defects are:

- *Gastrointestinal (duodenal atresia, abnormal visceral situs) = 12%–22% risk*
- *Omphalocele = 14%–40% risk*
- *Genitourinary (renal dysplasia, renal agenesis, hydronephrosis) = 5%–40% risk*
- *Central nervous system (hydrocephalus, agenesis of the corpus callosum, Dandy-Walker malformation) = 2%–15% risk*
- *Mediastinum (tracheoesophageal fistula, diaphragmatic hernia) = 10%–40% risk*
- *Vascular anomalies (single umbilical artery, persistent right umbilical vein) = No increased risk of cardiac defect when in isolation. When associated with other fetal anomalies, the risk for aneuploidy is 50%.*

▶ Drose JA: *Fetal Echocardiography*, 2nd edition. St. Louis, Saunders Elsevier, 2010, p 26.

▶ Woodward PJ, Kennedy A, Sohaey R, et al: *Diagnostic Imaging: Obstetrics*. Salt Lake City, AMIRSYS, 2005, ch 11, pp 10–13.

322. E. 90%–95%.

▶ Drose JA: *Fetal Echocardiography*, 2nd edition. St. Louis, Saunders Elsevier, 2010, p 282.

323. B. 17.1%.

▶ Drose JA: *Fetal Echocardiography*, 2nd edition. St. Louis, Saunders Elsevier, 2010, p 26.

324. C. Ectopia cordis.

325. A. Cardiomyopathy-induced arrhythmias.

Cardiomyopathy-induced dysrhythmia is the most common cause of nonimmune hydrops fetalis in North America. Dilated cardiomyopathies cause direct myocardial damage that may result in dysrhythmia, either brady- or tachydysrhythmia. See also answers 106 and 318.

▶ Drose JA: *Fetal Echocardiography*, 2nd edition. St. Louis, Saunders Elsevier, 2010, pp 295.

326. D. Maternal hyperthyroidism.

327. D. Transposition of the great arteries.

Because the great vessels are parallel to each other as they come off the heart, the defect must be transposition of the great arteries, supported by the patient's history of diabetes.

▶ Drose JA: *Fetal Echocardiography*, 2nd edition. St. Louis, Saunders Elsevier, 2010, p 26.

328. B. Type I diabetes mellitus.

▶ Drose JA: *Fetal Echocardiography*, 2nd edition. St. Louis, Saunders Elsevier, 2010, p 220.

329. A. Antibodies specific for SSA/Ro and SSB/La.

A mother who tests positive for these antibodies most likely has lupus, which can lead to fetal heart block.

▶ Drose JA: *Fetal Echocardiography*, 2nd edition. St. Louis, Saunders Elsevier, 2010, pp 26.

330. E. Both A (increased risk of cardiac defects) and B (increased risk of neural tube defects).

Cardiac and neural tube defects are more common in the fetuses of mothers with pregestational diabetes.

▶ Corrigan N, Brazil DP, McAuliffe F: Fetal cardiac effects of maternal hyperglycemia during pregnancy. Birth Defects Res A Clin Mol Teratol 85:523–530, 2009.

331. B. Complete heart block in the fetus.

Maternal lupus increases a fetus's risk for developing complete heart block. Fetal complete heart block occurs in approximately 5% of cases.

▶ Drose JA: *Fetal Echocardiography*, 2nd edition. St. Louis, Saunders Elsevier, 2010, p 26.

▶ Woodward PJ, Kennedy A, Sohaey R, et al: *Diagnostic Imaging: Obstetrics*. Salt Lake City, AMIRSYS, 2005, ch 6, p 77.

332. A. Human immunodeficiency virus (HIV).

HIV has NOT been shown to increase the risk of a developmental heart defect. Maternal infections that are known to cause direct myocardial damage, which may result in heart failure, include rubella, cytomegalovirus, parvovirus, and coxsackievirus.

▶ Drose JA: *Fetal Echocardiography*, 2nd edition. St. Louis, Saunders Elsevier, 2010, pp 293–298.

333. B. Hypertrophic cardiomyopathy.

334. A. Connective tissue disorder.

Circulation of maternal autoantibodies across the placenta increases the fetal risk for acquiring complete heart block to 1:60. If the anti-SSA/Ro antibody is present, the risk that the fetus will develop complete heart block is 1:20.

▶ Drose JA: *Fetal Echocardiography*, 2nd edition. St. Louis, Saunders Elsevier, 2010, p 309.

335. C. Rubella.

Maternal rubella infection has been associated with pulmonary atresia.

▶ Drose JA: *Fetal Echocardiography*, 2nd edition. St. Louis, Saunders Elsevier, 2010, p 179.

336. E. Both A (maternal diabetes) and D (hypertrophic cardiomyopathy).

Subvalvular aortic stenosis is the second most common type of aortic stenosis. It occurs more commonly in the pediatric patient but may occur in a fetus whose mother has poorly controlled diabetes. In these cases the fetus will have obstructive lesions of the left ventricle, resulting in hypertrophic cardiomyopathy.

▶ Drose JA: *Fetal Echocardiography*, 2nd edition. St. Louis, Saunders Elsevier, 2010, p 170.

337. D. Both A (rubella) and B (diabetes).

Subvalvular aortic stenosis commonly occurs with maternal diabetes, and supravalvular aortic stenosis is seen in cases of maternal rubella.

▶ Drose JA: *Fetal Echocardiography*, 2nd edition. St. Louis, Saunders Elsevier, 2010, p 175.

338. E. All of the above.

Hypertrophic cardiomyopathy is commonly associated with maternal diabetes, Noonan syndrome, glycogen storage disease, and twin-to-twin transfusion syndrome.

▶ Drose JA: *Fetal Echocardiography*, 2nd edition. St. Louis, Saunders Elsevier, 2010, pp 294–297.

339. C. Ventricular septal defect.

Ventricular septal defect has the highest recurrence rate and is the most teratogen-associated defect.

▶ Drose JA: *Fetal Echocardiography*, 2nd edition. St. Louis, Saunders Elsevier, 2010, p 105.

340. D. 25%–30%.

▶ Drose JA: *Fetal Echocardiography*, 1st edition. St. Louis, Saunders Elsevier, 1998, p 18.

341. A. Ductus arteriosus constriction.

Medicinal agents taken by the mother during pregnancy often cause ductal constriction in the fetus. The constriction may regress once the medicine is stopped.

342. E. All are true statements.

▸ Drose JA: *Fetal Echocardiography*, 2nd edition. St. Louis, Saunders Elsevier, 2010, p 18.

▸ Norton ME: Teratogen update: fetal effects of indomethacin administration during pregnancy. Teratology 56:282–292, 1997,
pp 282–292.

343. D. Nifedipine.

Nifedipine (trade names include Procardia and Adalat) is a medication prescribed to obstetric patients for preterm labor and contractions. It poses no risk to the developing fetus.

344. B. Ebstein anomaly.

Although the reasons are unknown, Ebstein anomaly appears with greater frequency in the infants of mothers who took lithium during early pregnancy.

▸ Agarwala BN, Hijazi ZM, Dearani J: Ebstein's anomaly of the tricuspid valve. UpToDate. Available at http://www.uptodate.com/contents/ebsteins-anomaly-of-the-tricuspid-valve.

▸ Drose JA: *Fetal Echocardiography*, 2nd edition. St. Louis, Saunders Elsevier, 2010, pp 198–199.

345. E. Maternal fever.

Maternal fever is associated with sinus tachycardia, NOT *premature atrial contractions (PACs). PACs may be associated with a redundant foramen ovale flap or maternal use of caffeine, cigarettes, or alcohol.*

▸ Drose JA: *Fetal Echocardiography*, 2nd edition. St. Louis, Saunders Elsevier, 2010, pp 307–308.

346. C. Congenital heart defects.

Approximately one-third of children with alcohol embryopathy will also have congenital cardiac problems, including a higher risk of ventricular septal defects, atrial septal defects, D-transposition, conotruncal heart defects, coarctation and hypoplastic aortic arch, shortened QT, and shortened left ventricular diameter. (The other choices are not the primary focus of fetal echocardiography.)

▸ Autti-Ramo I, Fagerlund A, Ervalahti N, et al: Fetal alcohol spectrum disorders in Finland: clinical delineation of 77 older children and adolescents. Am J Med Genet A 140:137–143, 2006.

▸ Carmichael SL, Shaw GM, Yang W, et al: Maternal periconceptional alcohol consumption and risk for conotruncal heart defects. Birth Defects Res A 67:875–878, 2003.

▸ Grewal J, Carmichael SL, Ma C, et al: Maternal periconceptional smoking and alcohol consumption and risk for select congenital anomalies. Birth Defects Res A 82:519–526, 2008.

▸ Krasemann T, Klingebiel S: Influence of chronic intrauterine exposure to alcohol on structurally normal hearts. Cardiol Young 17:185–188, 2007.

▸ Ornoy A, Ergaz Z: Alcohol abuse in pregnant women: effects on the fetus and newborn, mode of action and maternal treatment. Int J Environ Res Public Health 7:364–379, 2010.

▸ Tikkanen J, Heinonen OP: Risk factors for atrial septal defect. Eur J Epidemiol 8:509–515, 1992.

▸ Williams LJ, Correa A, Rasmussen S: Maternal lifestyle factors and risk for ventricular septal defects. Birth Defects Res A 70:59–64, 2004.

347. B. 4–8 weeks.

All major organ systems are formed between 4 and 8 weeks' gestation. This time period is when the organs begin to develop, referred to as organogenesis. *Any factors that interfere with development of these organ systems may cause faulty development.*

▸ Drose JA: *Fetal Echocardiography*, 2nd edition. St. Louis, Saunders Elsevier, 2010, p 1.

348. E. All of the above

> American Institute of Ultrasound in Medicine: AIUM practice parameter for the performance of fetal echocardiography. AIUM, 2013, p 1. Available at http://www.aium.org/resources/guidelines/fetalecho.pdf.

349. D. 25%–45%.

The incidence of extracardiac defects in a fetus diagnosed with a congenital heart defect is approximately 25%–45%. Some extracardiac malformations carry a high risk for association with heart defects, while others carry a low risk.

> Drose JA: *Fetal Echocardiography*, 2nd edition. St. Louis, Saunders Elsevier, 2010, p 26.

350. B. 35%.

The incidence of an abnormal karyotype in a fetus diagnosed with a congenital heart defect in utero would be 35%.

> Drose JA: *Fetal Echocardiography*, 2nd edition. St. Louis, Saunders Elsevier, 2010, p 19.

351. A. No increased risk.

An echogenic focus is an incidental finding and may be seen in approximately 3%–4% of all second trimester fetuses. In a low-risk patient, an echogenic focus is considered normal.

> Woodward PJ, Kennedy A, Sohaey R, et al: *Diagnostic Imaging: Obstetrics*. Salt Lake City, AMIRSYS, 2005, ch 6, p 6.

352. A. 11–14 weeks' gestation.

The optimal gestational age for performing a fetal nuchal translucency measurement is between 11 and 14 weeks' gestation. This is the time when the fetal crown-rump length (CRL) is between 45 and 84 mm. The success rate for an accurate measurement of the nuchal translucency decreases as CRL exceeds 84 mm; afterward shifting fetal position makes it more difficult to obtain the measurement.

> Nicolaides KD, Sebire NJ, Snijder RJM: *The 11–14 Week Scan: The Diagnosis of Fetal Abnormalities*. London, Parthenon, 1999, p 15.

353. C. 15%–30%.

Of fetuses with a serious congenital heart defect, between 15% and 30% have an increased nuchal translucency greater than 95% for gestational age. As nuchal translucency thickness increases, the risk for congenital heart defects increases as well.

> Ghi T, Huggon IC, Zosmer N, et al: Incidence of major structural cardiac defects associated with increased nuchal translucency but normal karyotype. Ultrasound Obstet Gynecol 18:610–614, 2001.

354. E. A (hypoplastic left heart syndrome), B (coarctation of the aorta), and C (aortic stenosis).

A, B, and C are all correct. Multiple types of cardiac defects are associated with an increased nuchal translucency, but there is an especially strong association with left-sided heart defects— commonly coarctation of the aorta, aortic stenosis/atresia, and hypoplastic left heart syndrome.

> Nicolaides KD, Sebire NJ, Snijder RJM: *The 11–14 Week Scan: The Diagnosis of Fetal Abnormalities*. London, Parthenon, 1999, pp 74–75.

355. E. A (4D sonography) and D (continuous-wave Doppler).

Both three- and four-dimensional sonography have been used to quantify fetal hemodynamic parameters (e.g., cardiac output) and to evaluate anatomic cardiac defects. Adjunctive Doppler modalities include tissue Doppler and continuous-wave Doppler.

> American Institute of Ultrasound in Medicine: AIUM practice parameter for the performance of fetal echocardiography. AIUM, 2013, p 6. Available at http://www.aium.org/resources/guidelines/fetalecho.pdf.

356. B. Spectral Doppler.

At mid gestation the normal fetal heart rate is 120–180 beats per minute. Documentation of the heart rate and rhythm should be made by measuring the cardiac cycle length with M-mode interrogation or spectral Doppler. If an abnormal heart rate (bradycardia or tachycardia) or irregular rhythm is documented, further assessment should be performed, according to the American Institute of Ultrasound in Medicine, "using either simultaneous Doppler sonography of the mitral inflow–aortic outflow or superior vena cava–ascending aorta, or by M-mode sonography of the atrium and ventricle to determine the underlying mechanism. An alternative approach using tissue Doppler sonography of the atrium and ventricle has also been described."

▶ American Institute of Ultrasound in Medicine: AIUM practice parameter for the performance of fetal echocardiography. AIUM, 2013. Available at http://www.aium.org/resources/guidelines/fetalecho.pdf.

▶ Baun J: *Ob/Gyn Sonography: An Illustrated Review*. Pasadena, CA, Davies Publishing, 2016, p 189.

357. C. Magnetic resonance imaging.

Magnetic resonance imaging (MRI) is a helpful adjunct to fetal ultrasound. MRI can depict subtle differences in fetal tissues to determine the exact location and size of a mass. MRI can also aid in assessment of surrounding structures and the effects of the mass on the cardiovascular system.

▶ Rychik J, Tian Z: *Fetal Cardiovascular Imaging: A Disease-Based Approach*. Philadelphia, Elsevier Saunders, 2012, pp 460–470.

358. E. A (MRI can better visualize the lung/liver tissue interfaces), B (MRI is helpful in determining heart displacement in the fetal thorax), and C (MRI helps determine liver position in the fetus).

Magnetic resonance imaging (MRI) is a helpful adjunct to fetal ultrasound when visualizing lung and liver tissue, determining heart location, and determining liver location. MRI can depict subtle differences in fetal tissues to determine the exact location and the size of a mass. MRI will depict lung/liver tissue interfaces that are sometimes difficult to distinguish using ultrasound. The position of the fetal liver is critical to determine for proper counseling. A liver that is in the fetal chest has a poorer prognosis and suggests an increased risk for pulmonary hypoplasia. MRI will also assess the surrounding structures and the effects of the mass on the cardiovascular system.

▶ Rychik J, Tian Z: *Fetal Cardiovascular Imaging: A Disease-Based Approach*. Philadelphia, Elsevier Saunders, 2012, pp 460–470.

359. B. Coarctation of the aorta.

The normal diameter of the aortic isthmus is 3.6 mm. The disproportion between the right and left ventricles suggests coarctation of the aorta.

▶ Drose JA: *Fetal Echocardiography*, 2nd edition. St. Louis, Saunders Elsevier, 2010, pp 186–193.

PART 5
Protocols

360. E. All of the above are true statements.

361. E. Both C (apical five-chamber view) and D (long-axis view of the aorta).

Persistent truncus arteriosus is very challenging to diagnose in utero. The apical and subcostal four-chamber views may appear normal. The five-chamber view and long-axis view of the aorta are two views used for diagnosing the characteristic single truncal valve overriding the interventricular septal defect.

▶ Drose JA: *Fetal Echocardiography*, 2nd edition. St. Louis, Saunders Elsevier, 2010, pp 226–228.

362. E. Both A (apical four-chamber view) and B (subcostal four-chamber view).

▶ Drose JA: *Fetal Echocardiography*, 2nd edition. St. Louis, Saunders Elsevier, 2010, p 123.

363. B. Short-axis view.

▶ Drose JA: *Fetal Echocardiography*, 2nd edition. St. Louis, Saunders Elsevier, 2010, pp 48, 125.

364. B. Subcostal four-chamber view.

In the subcostal four-chamber view, the ultrasound beam is perpendicular to the interventricular septum, therefore increasing the detection of conoventricular or perimembranous defects and decreasing dropout artifacts.

▶ Drose JA: *Fetal Echocardiography*, 2nd edition. St. Louis, Saunders Elsevier, 2010, pp 32–38.

365. D. Aortic wall continuity with the interventricular septum.

The aorta is located superior to the atrioventricular valves, so continuity of the aortic wall with the septum is NOT seen in the four-chamber view. The best view for this would be the long-axis view of the aorta. Refer to questions 17–25.

366. B. Subcostal four-chamber view.

The "apical four-chamber view" is also a correct answer when the probe is positioned above the fetal apex.

367. D. 40%–57%.

▶ Drose JA: *Fetal Echocardiography*, 2nd edition. St. Louis, Saunders Elsevier, 2010, p 28.

368. B. Parallel.

369. E. All of the above are considered standard views.

370. D. Left atrium.

The left atrium is the most posterior heart chamber and therefore the chamber closest to the fetal spine.

371. A. Long-axis view of the aorta.

372. C. Aortic arch.

The aortic arch has the classic "candy cane" appearance. The aortic arch should be seen exiting the fetal heart in the center of the fetal chest, giving rise to the head and neck vessels.

373. B. Long-axis view of the aorta.

In this view the aorta is elongated, allowing visualization of the left ventricular outflow tract (LVOT), mitral valve, and septum.

374. C. Left atrium, mitral valve, papillary muscle, right ventricle, and left ventricle.

The left atrium, mitral valve, papillary muscle, right ventricle, and left ventricle are all structures that should be seen in the long-axis view of the left heart. The pulmonic valve is NOT visualized because it lies superior to the aortic valve.

375. D. Pulmonary artery > aorta > superior vena cava.

In the normal heart, the pulmonary artery should be larger than the aorta because the right ventricle ejects the majority of blood flow, thereby increasing the diameter of the pulmonary artery compared to the aorta. The aorta is larger than the superior vena cava for the same reason. The higher the blood volume, the larger the diameter.

376. A. Cephalad, leftward, and posterior to the right ventricle.

377. A. 135-degree angle.

378. D. Anterior and superior.

379. E. Both A (where the aorta and pulmonary artery cross) and C (at the level of the semilunar valves).

The pulmonary artery and aorta cross at the level of the semilunar valves at approximately 135 degrees. The great vessels must cross each other at this level for the heart to be structurally normal.

380. E. Pulmonary veins.

381. D. Left ventricle.

In the short-axis view of the great vessels the left ventricle is located inferiorly. Therefore it is NOT visualized in this view.

▶ Drose JA: *Fetal Echocardiography*, 2nd edition. St. Louis, Saunders Elsevier, 2010, pp 46–52.

382. E. Short-axis view of the great vessels.

In the short-axis view of the great vessels the aortic root may be visualized. At this level the cusps of the aortic valve are seen in cross section. The aorta is seen as a "circle" in the center of the image with the pulmonary artery coursing around it.

▶ Drose JA: *Fetal Echocardiography*, 2nd edition. St. Louis, Saunders Elsevier, 2010, pp 46–49.

383. A. Fetal arrhythmias.

▶ Drose JA: *Fetal Echocardiography*, 2nd edition. St. Louis, Saunders Elsevier, 2010, pp 44–46, 60.

384. B. Short-axis view of the ventricles.

385. C. Pulmonary artery.

In the three-vessel view, the vessels are anteriorly/posteriorly related, NOT superiorly/inferiorly. Thus if you drew a line from anterior to posterior, the arrangement would be pulmonary artery > aorta > superior vena cava. The largest vessel would be the pulmonary artery, the aorta would be next largest, and the superior vena cava would be the smallest.

▶ Drose JA: *Fetal Echocardiography*, 2nd edition. St. Louis, Saunders Elsevier, 2010, pp 56–57.

386. B. Three-vessel view.

387. D. Both A (the ductus arteriosus has a "hockey stick" appearance) and C (the ductus arteriosus has a higher peak systolic velocity when compared to the aorta) are true.

The ductus arteriosus—the vessel that shunts blood flow between the fetal pulmonary trunk and proximal descending aorta—allows blood that has been oxygenated through the maternal lungs via the placenta to bypass the nonfunctioning fetal lungs and enter the fetal circulation. The ductus

arteriosus has a "hockey stick" appearance on echocardiography as opposed to the "candy cane" appearance of the aortic arch. The ductus arteriosus is narrower than the aorta and therefore flow within it has a higher velocity.

▶ Drose JA: *Fetal Echocardiography*, 2nd edition. St. Louis, Saunders Elsevier, 2010, pp 53–54.

388. A. Mitral valve.

▶ Drose JA: *Fetal Echocardiography*, 2nd edition. St. Louis, Saunders Elsevier, 2010, pp 53–54.

389. A. The diameter of the superior vena cava is larger than that of the inferior vena cava.

The diameter of the superior vena cava should be slightly smaller than that of the inferior vena cava because there is more blood flow returning from the body than the head.

▶ Drose JA: *Fetal Echocardiography*, 2nd edition. St. Louis, Saunders Elsevier, 2010, pp 56–59.

390. B. Premature atrial contraction.

The flow seen below the baseline is atrial filling, and ventricular ejection is represented above the baseline. Premature atrial contraction is manifested on the waveform as the absence of an E-wave component in the atrial activation. There is ventricular ejection following the premature atrial contraction.

391. C. Blocked premature atrial contraction.

There is an early atrial contraction with atrial conduction blocked to the ventricle; the waveform to which the arrow is pointing represents a blocked premature atrial contraction.

392. D. M-mode.

M-mode displays depth (on the vertical axis) versus time (on the horizontal axis). With M-mode (motion mode) the sound beam is in a fixed position and the sound pulse travels down the same path repeatedly over time as the object of interrogation moves. M-mode is used mainly to demonstrate movement of cardiac structures.

▶ Kremkau FW: *Sonography: Principles and Instruments*, 9th edition. St. Louis, Elsevier, 2016, pp 105–106.

393. A. M-mode.

In compliance with ALARA standards, documentation of embryonic cardiac activity in a healthy first trimester pregnancy is accomplished using M-mode rather than spectral Doppler, which is associated with a higher level of acoustic output.

▶ American Institute of Ultrasound in Medicine: AIUM practice parameter for the performance of obstetric ultrasound examinations. AIUM, 2013, p 12. Available at http://www.aium.org/resources/guidelines/fetalecho.pdf.

▶ Baun J: *Ob/Gyn Sonography: An Illustrated Review*. Pasadena, CA, Davies Publishing, 2016, pp 165, 307.

394. B. M-mode tracing.

395. E. Both B (subcostal four-chamber view) and D (short-axis view of the left ventricle) are acceptable.

To measure the interventricular septum and the ventricular dimension, the M-mode must be placed perpendicular to the sound beam.

396. D. M-mode.

M-mode stands for "motion mode" and displays a single scan line of information over time. Therefore it can be used to document the movement of the fetal heart. It is a form of B-mode (brightness mode), not Doppler. B-color is colorization of B-mode pixels.

▶ Baun J: *Ob/Gyn Sonography: An Illustrated Review*. Pasadena, CA, Davies Publishing, 2016, p 444.

397. C. Tachycardic.

A normal second trimester fetal heart rate is between 100 and 180 beats per minute (bpm). The M-mode image identifies the fetal heart rate as 184 bpm, which is in the tachycardic range.

▶ Baun J: *Ob/Gyn Sonography: An Illustrated Review*. Pasadena, CA, Davies Publishing, 2016, p 189.

398. A. Complete heart block.

The waveform documents dissociation between the atrial and ventricular rates. The atrial rate is normal at 140 beats per minute (bpm), while the ventricular rate is slow at 76 bpm.

399. C. >0.5.

Normal heart circumference is less than 50% (0.5) of the thoracic circumference. A heart circumference to thoracic circumference ratio that is greater than 50% of the thorax is considered cardiomegaly.

400. C. Pulmonic valve; normal.

In this image of the pulmonary artery the calipers are measuring the pulmonic valve. This measurement is in the normal range for a 28-week fetus. The normal range is 5.0–7.0 mm.

▶ Drose JA: *Fetal Echocardiography*, 2nd edition. St. Louis, Saunders Elsevier, 2010, pp 43–48.

401. D. 1:2.

The atria should be half the size of the ventricles when measured from the anterior to the posterior wall. When the examiner is visually assessing the chamber size, two atria when placed on top of each other should fit in one ventricle.

402. B. Pericardial effusion.

Pericardial effusion is a fluid collection in the pericardial space surrounding the heart.

▶ Woodward PJ, Kennedy A, Sohaey R, et al: *Diagnostic Imaging: Obstetrics*. Salt Lake City, AMIRSYS, 2005, ch 6, pp 11–12.

403. B. Hypoechoic rim of fluid less than 2 mm.

Pericardial effusion is diagnosed when the fluid collection in the pericardial space surrounding the heart measures more than 2 mm. When the fluid collection exceeds 2 mm it is considered pathologic.

▶ Woodward PJ, Kennedy A, Sohaey R, et al: *Diagnostic Imaging: Obstetrics*. Salt Lake City, AMIRSYS, 2005, ch 6, pp 11–12.

PART 6
Physics and Instrumentation

404. A. Frequency.

Frequency *is defined as the number of cycles in a wave produced in one second. The higher the frequency, the faster the ultrasound energy will be absorbed. The* wavelength *is the distance traveled by sound in one cycle. It is inversely proportional to the frequency. The smaller the wavelength, the higher the frequency. Higher-frequency sound waves result in less tissue penetration but higher resolution, whereas lower-frequency sound waves are better at penetrating to deeper focal areas, but with lower resolution. A 12 MHz transducer will emit sound waves that penetrate tissue less deeply than those of a 2 MHz transducer.*

▸ Kremkau FW: *Sonography: Principles and Instruments*, 9th edition. St. Louis, Elsevier, 2016, pp 15, 27–28.

405. E. Bone.

Absorption varies greatly in different tissues. The ability to absorb energy in fluids is poor, but it is very high in bone. (Another way to ask this question is, "Which of these types of tissue transmits sound the fastest?")

406. D. Time gain compensation.

Time gain compensation *(TGC), also called* depth gain compensation *(DGC) or simply* compensation, *adjusts for the varying strengths of echoes from reflectors at different depths. As the beam travels, the signal strength decreases due to attenuation. Therefore, when echoes are reflected from structures farther away from the transducer, the returning signals will be weaker than those reflected from structures closer to the transducer. TGC "compensates" for this phenomenon by increasing the brightness of distant echoes to achieve a level of brightness on the image that is "equalized" to represent various structures' echogenicity without the effects of attenuation.*

▸ Kremkau FW: *Sonography: Principles and Instruments*, 9th edition. St. Louis, Elsevier, 2016, pp 185–187.

▸ Penny SM, Fox TB, Godwin CH: *Exam Review for Ultrasound: Sonography Principles and Instrumentation*. Philadelphia, Wolters/Kluwer, 2011, p 76.

407. B. Pulse repetition frequency (PRF).

Pulse repetition frequency *(PRF) is the number of pulses of sound produced in 1 second. Think of bouncing a ball against a wall. If you are 1 foot away from the wall, the ball would return quickly and therefore the rate of return would be high. As the distance between you and the wall decreases, PRF increases. If you are 15 feet from the wall, the time it takes the ball to return to you increases—that is, the rate at which the ball returns to you in the same period of time is much lower. It is the same with ultrasound: As the depth increases, the PRF decreases.*

▸ Kremkau FW: *Sonography: Principles and Instruments*, 9th edition. St. Louis, Elsevier, 2016, pp 19–20.

408. E. All of these statements are true except A.

▸ Kremkau FW: *Sonography: Principles and Instruments*, 9th edition. St. Louis, Elsevier, 2016, pp 161–163.

409. D. A (adjust the focal zone closer to the apex) and B (increase frequency).

410. A. Near field.

411. B. As low as [is] reasonably achievable.

ALARA—"as low as reasonably achievable"—is the principle that all sonographers must follow to practice safe scanning procedures and safe operation of the ultrasound equipment. The sonographer must use the lowest reasonable power levels and exposure ("dwell time") necessary to achieve a high-quality image and technical examination.

▸ American Institute of Ultrasound in Medicine: AIUM practice parameter for the performance of fetal echocardiography. AIUM, 2013, p 7. Available at http://www.aium.org/resources/guidelines/fetalecho.pdf.

▸ Kremkau FW: *Sonography: Principles and Instruments*, 9th edition. St. Louis, Elsevier, 2016, pp 221, 235.

412. A. Cavitation.

     Cavitation *is the action of an acoustic fluid within a field to generate bubbles. There are two types, stable and transient.* Stable cavitation *produces bubbles that do not rupture.* Transient cavitation *generates larger bubbles that may rupture, cause a shock wave, and generate heat in the tissue.*

     ▸ Kremkau FW: *Sonography: Principles and Instruments*, 9th edition. St. Louis, Elsevier, 2016, pp 221, 231–232.

     ▸ Penny SM, Fox TB, Godwin CH: *Exam Review for Ultrasound: Sonography Principles and Instrumentation*. Philadelphia, Wolters/Kluwer, 2011, p 156.

413. E. A (thermal effects) and C (mechanical effects).

     Thermal effects *cause a rise in body temperature in tissues due to absorption of energy, which is transformed into heat.* Mechanical effects *result in cavitation.* Cavitation *is the interaction of ultrasound waves and gas bubbles in the tissues.*

     ▸ Kremkau FW: *Sonography: Principles and Instruments*, 9th edition. St. Louis, Elsevier, 2016, pp 220–233.

414. C. <2.0 degrees Celsius.

     An increase in temperature that exceeds 2 degrees Celsius is considered significant. Thermal effects from diagnostic ultrasound beams are generally considered safe (i.e., have no adverse effects) at even higher levels, depending on exposure times. However, the probability of adverse thermal effects increases with the duration of the increased temperature, and adult tissues generally tolerate temperature increases better than fetal or neonatal tissues.

     ▸ Kremkau FW: *Sonography: Principles and Instruments*, 9th edition. St. Louis, Elsevier, 2016, pp 224–227.

415. C. Keeping both output power and exposure time as low as reasonably achievable.

     ▸ American Institute of Ultrasound in Medicine: AIUM practice parameter for the performance of fetal echocardiography. AIUM, 2013, p 7. Available at http://www.aium.org/resources/guidelines/fetalecho.pdf.

416. A. Between the transducer surface and the focal zone.

417. C. 5–7 MHz.

     Fetal imaging studies performed from the anterior abdominal wall can usually use frequencies of 5.0 MHz or higher. Axial and lateral resolution and depth of penetration are dependent on ultrasound frequency, maternal body habitus, gestational age, and amniotic fluid volume. The higher the frequency, the higher the resolution but the lower the depth of penetration.

     ▸ American Institute of Ultrasound in Medicine: AIUM practice parameter for the performance of fetal echocardiography. AIUM, 2013, p 6. Available at http://www.aium.org/resources/guidelines/fetalecho.pdf.

     ▸ Drose JA: *Fetal Echocardiography*, 2nd edition. St. Louis, Saunders Elsevier, 2010, p 16.

418. C. Focal zone.

     The sound field is composed of a narrow field called the near field, *a far field that diverges as it gets farther from the transducer, and a* focal zone (or focal point) *where the sound beam is at its narrowest.*

419. A. Increase pulse repetition frequency (PRF).

     The PRF was set at 0.9 kHz. Increasing the PRF will decrease the number of pulses transmitted per second, eliminating the noise and scatter of the ultrasound frequencies.

420. E. All of the above.

421. B. Attenuation.

     Shadowing occurs when sound travels through an area of higher attenuation (such as fetal ribs or a gallstone) compared with the area of surrounding tissue—attenuation is higher in bones than in soft tissues. The shadowing artifact is useful because it helps with the identification of the gallstone.

     ▸ Kremkau FW: *Sonography: Principles and Instruments*, 9th edition. St. Louis, Elsevier, 2016, p 27.

     ▸ Penny SM, Fox TB, Godwin CH: *Exam Review for Ultrasound: Sonography Principles and Instrumentation*. Philadelphia, Wolters/Kluwer, 2011, p 155.

422. B. Reverberation artifact.

Reverberation artifact occurs when the ultrasound wave impinges on a strong reflector with a large surface area in the near field. Sound waves are reflected and return as echoes. The sound waves oscillate back and forth between the probe and the reflector. This object will appear to be displayed several times at several different depths.

▶ Kremkau FW: *Sonography: Principles and Instruments*, 9th edition. St. Louis, Elsevier, 2016, pp 81–82.

▶ Penny SM, Fox TB, Godwin CH: *Exam Review for Ultrasound: Sonography Principles and Instrumentation*. Philadelphia, Wolters/Kluwer, 2011, p 84.

423. B. Shadowing.

424. D. They represent multiple reflections of the same object.

Reverberation artifact, not shadowing, results in the same object displayed several times at different depths.

▶ Kremkau FW: *Sonography: Principles and Instruments*, 9th edition. St. Louis, Elsevier, 2016, pp 81–82, 193–196.

425. E. All of these adjustments will eliminate this artifact.

426. E. A (fetal rib shadows) and C (a poor acoustic window).

427. B. Dropout artifact.

428. B. The transmitted sound beam is parallel to the septum.

429. C. Shadowing artifact caused by fetal ribs.

The shadowing artifact is displayed as multiple equally spaced echoes transmitted into the far field and is caused by bright reflectors—in this case fetal ribs—in the near field.

430. A. Speckle.

Attenuation *is a decrease in the amplitude, power, and intensity of the sound beam as sound travels through tissue.* Side-lobe artifacts *are caused by extraneous sound that is not found along the primary beam path; they occur with single-element transducers.* Mirror-image artifacts *are the result of sound bouncing off a strong reflector, which causes a structure to appear on both sides of the reflector.* Enhancement *is an artifact caused by sound passing through an area of lower attenuation.*

▶ Penny SM, Fox TB, Godwin CH: *Exam Review for Ultrasound: Sonography Principles and Instrumentation*. Philadelphia, Wolters/Kluwer, 2011, p 199.

431. D. Wall filter.

Other names for the wall filter are wall-motion filter, high-pass filter, *and* wall-thump filter. *For cardiac imaging, a high* wall-filter *setting is used to counteract the movement of the myocardial tissue and valves.*

▶ Penny SM, Fox TB, Godwin CH: *Exam Review for Ultrasound: Sonography Principles and Instrumentation*. Philadelphia, Wolters/Kluwer, 2011, p 125.

432. A. Aliasing.

The waveform has exceeded the maximum frequency available, therefore reaching the Nyquist limit. When the Nyquist limit is exceeded, the result is an aliasing artifact. The maximum Doppler frequency is reflected in the opposite direction. Refer to answer 436.

▶ Kremkau FW: *Sonography: Principles and Instruments*, 9th edition. St. Louis, Elsevier, 2016, pp 196–200.

433. D. Decreasing overall gain.

Overall gain will have no effect on the Doppler tracing.

434. E. Wall filter.

The umbilical artery waveform does not completely fill the envelope. The low-level echoes near the baseline were rejected and only the high-frequency echoes were displayed. Note the absence of signal near the baseline. For this image the wall filter was set too high.

▶ Penny SM, Fox TB, Godwin CH: *Exam Review for Ultrasound: Sonography Principles and Instrumentation*. Philadelphia, Wolters/Kluwer, 2011, p 125.

435. D. Decrease color gain.

436. E. Aliasing.

The correct answer, aliasing, *occurs when the frequency shift exceeds one-half of the pulse repetition frequency. This produces a wraparound of the Doppler signal whereby positive shifts are displayed as negative shifts. In color Doppler aliasing displays artifactually as bright, turbulent flow, and in spectral Doppler as profiles that "wrap around" the displayed scale. By contrast,* reflection *occurs when the sound beam strikes an interface at a 90-degree angle and there exists a large impedance difference between the two tissues.* Refraction *is the redirection of the transmitted sound beam.* Compensation—*also referred to as* time gain compensation *(TGC) or* depth gain compensation *(DGC)—is the parameter that adjusts for the varying strengths of echoes from reflectors at different depths.* Demodulation *processes the signal to make it easier for the machine to handle.*

437. C. Adjust the baseline.

438. A. Color Doppler imaging.

Color Doppler imaging *(also called* color flow imaging*) displays blood flow velocity and direction (or other tissue motion) by assigning color to frequency-shifted echoes.*

▶ Kremkau FW: *Sonography: Principles and Instruments*, 9th edition. St. Louis, Elsevier, 2016, pp 144–156.

439. E. All of the above.

Color Doppler imaging *assigns color to Doppler-shifted echoes to represent flow velocity, flow direction, and flow disturbances—i.e., based on the differences between transmitted and reflected frequencies.*

▶ Kremkau FW: *Sonography: Principles and Instruments*, 9th edition. St. Louis, Elsevier, 2016, p 144.

440. E. All of the above.

Because Color Doppler imaging can display information on blood flow velocity and direction, it helps locate blood flow disturbances and turbulence.

441. E. Both C (antegrade flow) and D (continuous flow).

The flow across the ductus arteriosus is a continuous forward, antegrade flow without any signs of reversal/retrograde flow. The color box shows the flow leaving the right ventricle and flowing away from the transducer in the normal antegrade fashion.

442. B. Aliasing.

443. D. Antegrade flow across the aortic arch.

444. B. Color Doppler.

445. B. Flow is from the right ventricle to the left ventricle.

446. A. Decrease the pulse repetition frequency (PRF).

Scale *is another term for PRF.*

447. B. Power Doppler.

448. E. All of the above are benefits.

Power Doppler imaging (also known as Doppler-power display *or* color power Doppler*) overcomes some of the limitations of conventional color Doppler imaging, such as angle dependence, aliasing, and difficulty in separating background noise from true flow in slow-flow states. Power Doppler sonography is valuable in detecting flow in low-flow states, producing better edge definition and depiction of continuity of flow when optimal Doppler angles cannot be obtained. Power Doppler is a "nondirectional" flow Doppler, as opposed to "directional-dependent flow" with standard color Doppler. See also answer 450.*

▶ Kremkau FW: *Sonography: Principles and Instruments*, 9th edition. St. Louis, Elsevier, 2016, p 156.

449. E. None of the above.

Power Doppler cannot display velocity-determined functions.

450. E. None of these functions is available with power Doppler.

Power Doppler assigns color to represent the Doppler shift power (strength) values, NOT *the Doppler shift frequency values. Baseline and pulse repetition frequency (scale) are velocity-dependent functions. Power Doppler is used independently of velocity. Power Doppler is "nondirectional"—it does not depict direction of flow—whereas standard color Doppler imaging is directional, depicting flow by means of color coding. Power Doppler imaging overcomes some of the limitations of conventional color Doppler ultrasound, such as angle dependence, aliasing, and difficulty in separating background noise from true flow in slow-flow states. Power Doppler sonography is valuable in detecting flow in low-flow states, producing better edge definition and depiction of continuity of flow when optimal Doppler angles cannot be obtained.*

▶ Kremkau FW: *Sonography: Principles and Instruments*, 9th edition. St. Louis, Elsevier, 2016, p 156.

451. C. Atrial systole.

452. C. Biphasic, 20–40 cm/sec.

453. E. Both B (congestive heart failure) and C (volume overload).

▶ Allan L, Hornberger L, Sharland G: *Textbook of Fetal Cardiology*. London, Greenwich Medical Media, 2000, p 570.

454. E. All of the above.

455. C. Triphasic flow.

456. E. All of the above.

457. E. Both A (reduced A wave toward the baseline) and B (reversed flow of the A wave during atrial contraction).

Both reduced A wave toward the baseline and reversed flow of the A wave during atrial contraction would signify an abnormal flow in the ductus venosus.

▶ Drose JA: *Fetal Echocardiography*, 2nd edition. St. Louis, Saunders Elsevier, 2010, p 65.

458. E. All of the above.

459. D. E wave.

Caliper 1 marks the E wave, rapid ventricular filling.

460. A. A wave.

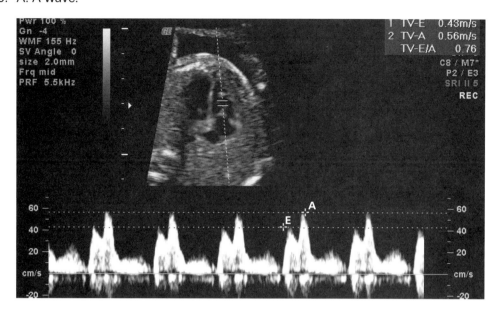

Normal blood flow through the mitral and tricuspid valves takes place during diastole. Pulsed-wave Doppler displays two wave peaks for these valves: at ventricular filling during early diastole, known as the E wave or E point, and at ventricular filling during atrial systole, known as the A point or A wave. The greater part of diastolic filling normally occurs during atrial systole and displays on the waveform as the "taller" A wave.

▶ Drose JA: *Fetal Echocardiography*, 2nd edition. St. Louis, Saunders Elsevier, 2010, pp 33, 63–64.

461. E. A (by placing the sample volume gate distal to the tricuspid valve), B (by maintaining the angle of insonation at 0 degrees), and C (by setting the sample volume size at 2 mm).

462. B. Pulsed-wave Doppler.

The high output power of pulsed-wave Doppler contraindicates its use for screening purposes, particularly in the first trimester of a pregnancy. See answers 393 and 411.

463. E. >140 cm per second.

A peak systolic velocity in the ductus arteriosus that exceeds 140 cm per second has been reported in cases of ductal constriction.

▶ Drose JA: *Fetal Echocardiography*, 2nd edition. St. Louis, Saunders Elsevier, 2010, p 55.

PART 7
Managing Medical Emergencies

464. A. Vasovagal response.

465. A. Roll her onto her left side, right side up.

Supine hypotensive syndrome is caused by excessive pressure on the inferior vena cava (IVC), known as the vasovagal response, *which leads to a decrease in blood pressure and thus a feeling of faintness and nausea. These symptoms are usually relieved by rolling the patient onto her left side, right side up, known as the* left lateral decubitus position. *This relieves pressure on the IVC.*

466. C. >5 mm.

Absence of cardiac activity in fetuses greater than 5 mm long indicates fetal demise and should be reported immediately to the supervising physician.

▶ Woodward PJ, Kennedy A, Sohaey R, et al: *Diagnostic Imaging: Obstetrics.* Salt Lake City, AMIRSYS, 2005, ch 6, p 2.

467. B. L-transposition of the great arteries.

L-transposition is NOT *a ductal-dependent lesion due to the inversion of the ventricles. The blood flow postnatally is "corrected" (in series). The right ventricle is able to supply the systemic circulation postnatally. All the other lesions may require medication to keep the ductus arteriosus patent after delivery.*

468. B. Prostaglandin E.

469. E. All these associated complications make close surveillance necessary.

470. A. Complete heart block.

Approximately 50% of fetuses with complete heart block have complex structural heart defects, usually atrioventricular septal defects, which have a high association with polysplenia and Down syndrome. Hydrops is also common in cases of complete heart block. See also answer 106.

▶ Drose JA: *Fetal Echocardiography,* 2nd edition. St. Louis, Saunders Elsevier, 2010, p 309.

471. C. Maternal digoxin therapy.

If a fetus has supraventricular tachycardia with no signs of hydrops or decompensation, medical therapy is warranted. Digoxin is the drug given to the mother of the fetus to manage fetal supraventricular tachycardia.

▶ Drose JA: *Fetal Echocardiography,* 2nd edition. St. Louis, Saunders Elsevier, 2010, pp 318–320.

472. D. Immediate delivery.

In cases of supraventricular tachycardia with fetal hydrops and signs of decompensation, immediate delivery is recommended if the pregnancy is at term.

▶ Drose JA: *Fetal Echocardiography,* 2nd edition. St. Louis, Saunders Elsevier, 2010, pp 318–320.

▶ Strasburger JF, Cheulkar B, Wichman HJ: Perinatal arrhythmias: diagnosis and management. Clin Perinatol 34:627–652, 2007.

473. A. Hypertrophic cardiomyopathy.

Twin-to-twin transfusion syndrome may result in high-output failure induced by volume overload. Mono-chorionic twins share placental circulation. Blood is transferred from the donor twin through the placenta to the recipient twin. This causes the donor twin to become anemic and the recipient twin to have volume overload. This leads to hyperviscosity and polycythemia, medial thickening throughout the pulmonary and systemic vascular beds, and evolution of biventricular hypertrophy.

▶ Drose JA: *Fetal Echocardiography,* 2nd edition. St. Louis, Saunders Elsevier, 2010, pp 296–297.

474. E. All of the above.

Fetal anemia is a cause of high-output failure leading to a form of dilated cardiomyopathy. Twin-to-twin transfusion syndrome (TTTS) and arteriovenous malformations (AVMs) cause volume overload as a result of massive arterial venous shunting.

▸ Drose JA: *Fetal Echocardiography*, 2nd edition. St. Louis, Saunders Elsevier, 2010, pp 59–60, 62, 293–296.

475. D. Both A (the lesion must have a poor prognosis with standard therapy) and B (fetal intervention will slow or halt progression of the lesion).

Fetal cardiac intervention can be considered even when there is a standard postnatal therapy if (1) the abnormality is progressive such that prenatal intervention promises to slow or halt this progression, AND (2) the abnormality has a poor prognosis with standard postnatal therapy.

▸ Drose JA: *Fetal Echocardiography*, 2nd edition. St. Louis, Saunders Elsevier, 2010, p 338.

PART 9

Application for CME Credit

***Fetal Echocardiography Review*, 2nd Edition**

This continuing medical educational (CME) activity is approved for 12 hours of credit by the Society of Diagnostic Medical Sonography. This credit may be applied as follows:

▸ Sonographers and technologists may apply these hours toward the CME requirements of the ARDMS, ARRT, and/or CCI, as well as to the CME requirements of most other organizations that may accredit your facility.

▸ SDMS-approved credit is not applicable toward the AMA Physician's Recognition Award but may be applicable to the CME requirements for physicians associated with accredited ultrasound facilities. Be sure to confirm requirements with the pertinent organizations.

▸ If you have any questions whatsoever about CME requirements that affect you, please contact the responsible organization directly for current information. CME requirements can and sometimes do change.

Objectives of This Activity

Upon completion of this educational activity, you will be able to:

1. Describe and explain embryologic development of the fetal heart.

2. Identify and explain why and when fetal echocardiography is performed.

3. Explain the incidence of and factors involved in congenital heart disease.

4. Describe the standard sonographic views of the fetal heart.

5. Identify, describe, and explain normal anatomy and physiology of the fetal heart.

6. Describe and explain structural anomalies of the fetal heart.

7. Describe and explain dysrhythmias of the fetal heart.

8. Describe, identify, and explain acquired and miscellaneous pathology of the fetal heart.

How to Obtain CME Credit

To apply for credit, please do all of the following:

1. Read and study the mock exam questions.

2. Photocopy and complete the following applicant information page, evaluation questionnaire (you grade us!), and CME answer sheet.

3. Return the completed forms together with payment of the administrative processing fee of $39.50 (if you are the book's original purchaser) or $49.50 (for borrowers) to the following address:

Davies Publishing, Inc.
CME Coordinator
32 South Raymond Avenue, Suite 4
Pasadena, California 91105-1961

You can also fax the appropriate pages to 626-792-5308 and pay by credit card. We grade quizzes within 24 business hours of receipt and will email your certificate to the email address you provide in your application form. Questions? Please call us at 626-792-3046.

4. If more than one person will be applying for credit, be sure to photocopy the applicant information, evaluation form, and CME quiz so that you always have the original on hand for use.

Applicant Information

Fetal Echocardiography Review, 2nd Edition

Name _____ Date of Birth _____

Your degrees and credentials _____

Address _____

City/State/ZIP _____

Telephone _____ Email (required) _____

ARDMS # _____ ARRT # _____ CCI # _____

SDMS # _____ Sonography Canada# _____

Payment Information
❏ I purchased this book new (fee is $39.50).
❏ I borrowed the book or purchased it used (fee is $49.50).

Credit Card # _____ Exp Date _____ 3- or 4-digit code _____

Name and address on credit card (if different from above)

_____

_____

_____

Signature and date certifying your completion of the activity:

_____

NOTE: The original purchaser of this CME activity is entitled to submit this CME application for an administrative fee of $39.50. Please enclose a check payable to Davies Publishing, Inc., or include credit card information with your application. Others may also submit applications for CME credits by completing the activity for an administrative fee of $49.50. The CME administrative fee helps to defray the cost of processing, evaluating, and maintaining a record of your application and the credit you earn. Fees may change without notice. For the current fee, call us at 626-792-3046, email us at **cme@daviespublishing.com**, or write to us at the aforementioned address. We will be happy to help!

Answer Sheet

Fetal Echocardiography Review, 2nd Edition

Circle the correct answer below and return this sheet to Davies Publishing, Inc. Passing criterion is 70%. Applicant may not have more than 3 attempts to pass.

1. A B C D E	31. A B C D E	61. A B C D E	91. A B C D E
2. A B C D E	32. A B C D E	62. A B C D E	92. A B C D E
3. A B C D E	33. A B C D E	63. A B C D E	93. A B C D E
4. A B C D E	34. A B C D E	64. A B C D E	94. A B C D E
5. A B C D E	35. A B C D E	65. A B C D E	95. A B C D E
6. A B C D E	36. A B C D E	66. A B C D E	96. A B C D E
7. A B C D E	37. A B C D E	67. A B C D E	97. A B C D E
8. A B C D E	38. A B C D E	68. A B C D E	98. A B C D E
9. A B C D E	39. A B C D E	69. A B C D E	99. A B C D E
10. A B C D E	40. A B C D E	70. A B C D E	100. A B C D E
11. A B C D E	41. A B C D E	71. A B C D E	101. A B C D E
12. A B C D E	42. A B C D E	72. A B C D E	102. A B C D E
13. A B C D E	43. A B C D E	73. A B C D E	103. A B C D E
14. A B C D E	44. A B C D E	74. A B C D E	104. A B C D E
15. A B C D E	45. A B C D E	75. A B C D E	105. A B C D E
16. A B C D E	46. A B C D E	76. A B C D E	106. A B C D E
17. A B C D E	47. A B C D E	77. A B C D E	107. A B C D E
18. A B C D E	48. A B C D E	78. A B C D E	108. A B C D E
19. A B C D E	49. A B C D E	79. A B C D E	109. A B C D E
20. A B C D E	50. A B C D E	80. A B C D E	110. A B C D E
21. A B C D E	51. A B C D E	81. A B C D E	111. A B C D E
22. A B C D E	52. A B C D E	82. A B C D E	112. A B C D E
23. A B C D E	53. A B C D E	83. A B C D E	113. A B C D E
24. A B C D E	54. A B C D E	84. A B C D E	114. A B C D E
25. A B C D E	55. A B C D E	85. A B C D E	115. A B C D E
26. A B C D E	56. A B C D E	86. A B C D E	116. A B C D E
27. A B C D E	57. A B C D E	87. A B C D E	117. A B C D E
28. A B C D E	58. A B C D E	88. A B C D E	118. A B C D E
29. A B C D E	59. A B C D E	89. A B C D E	119. A B C D E
30. A B C D E	60. A B C D E	90. A B C D E	120. A B C D E

Evaluation—You Grade Us!

Please let us know what you think of *Fetal Echocardiography Review, 2nd Edition*. Participating in this quality survey is a requirement for CME applicants, and it benefits future readers by ensuring that current readers are satisfied and, if not, that their comments and opinions are heard and taken into account.

1. Why did you purchase *Fetal Echocardiography Review*? (Circle your primary reason.)

   Registry review   Course text   Clinical reference   CME activity

2. Have you used *Fetal Echocardiography Review* for other reasons, too? (Circle all that apply.)

   Registry review   Course text   Clinical reference   CME activity

3. To what extent did *Fetal Echocardiography Review* meet its stated objectives and your needs? (Circle one.)

   Greatly   Moderately   Minimally   Insignificantly

4. The content of *Fetal Echocardiography Review* was (circle one):

   Just right   Too basic   Too advanced

5. The quality of the questions, explanations, illustrations, and case examples was mainly (circle one):

   Excellent   Good   Fair   Poor

6. The manner in which *Fetal Echocardiography Review* presents the material is mainly (circle one):

   Excellent   Good   Fair   Poor

7. If you used *Fetal Echocardiography Review* to prepare for the registry exam, did you also use other materials or take any exam-preparation courses?

   No   Yes   (please specify what materials and courses)

   _____

   _____

   _____

8. If you used *Fetal Echocardiography Review* for a course, please list the course name, the instructor's name, the name of the school or program, and any other textbooks you may have used:

   Course/instructor/school or program _____

   _____

   _____

9. What did you like best about *Fetal Echocardiography Review*?

   _____

   _____

   _____

10. What did you like least about *Fetal Echocardiography Review*?

    _____

    _____

    _____

11. If you used *Fetal Echocardiography Review* to prepare for your registry exam in fetal echocardiography, did you pass?

    Yes   No   Haven't yet taken it

12. May we quote any of your comments in our catalogs or promotional material?

    Yes   No   Further comment:

    _____

    _____

    _____

    _____

    _____

    _____

    _____

    _____

    _____

    _____

    _____

    _____

    _____

    _____

    _____

CME Quiz

Fetal Echocardiography Review, 2nd Edition

Please answer the following questions after you have completed the CME activity. There is one best answer for each question. Circle it on the answer sheet. The passing criterion is 70%. The applicant can make no more than 3 attempts to pass and earn credit.

1. Which one of the following conditions is NOT a ductal-dependent lesion?
   A. L-transposition of the great arteries
   B. Univentricular heart
   C. Severe pulmonic stenosis
   D. D-transposition of the great arteries
   E. Coarctation of the aorta

2. At what gestational age does organogenesis occur?
   A. 4–8 weeks
   B. 8–10 weeks
   C. 10–12 weeks
   D. 3–6 weeks
   E. 0–3 weeks

3. What structure or structures should be seen entering the left atrium when you are scanning through the normal fetal heart in the subcostal four-chamber heart view?
   A. Coronary sinus
   B. Inferior vena cava
   C. Superior vena cava
   D. Pulmonary veins
   E. Aortic arch

4. Which of the following characterizes the left atrium?
   A. It has a broad-based appendage.
   B. It has a finger-like, thin appendage.
   C. It contains the sinoatrial node.
   D. It receives the superior and inferior venae cavae.
   E. All of the above.

5. What causes embryologic pulmonic stenosis?
   A. Abnormal intracardiac blood flow
   B. Abnormal targeted growth
   C. Cell death abnormality
   D. Extracellular matrix abnormality
   E. Tissue-migration abnormality

6. Which of the following conditions is NOT generally associated with hypertrophic cardiomyopathies?

   A. Maternal diabetes
   B. Noonan syndrome
   C. Fetal anemia
   D. Glycogen storage disease
   E. Twin-to-twin transfusion syndrome

7. What is the normal range for the E/A ratio?

   A. Constant at 1.5
   B. 0.5–1.0
   C. 1.1–1.5
   D. 1.5–2.0
   E. 2.0–3.0

8. You are measuring the fetal pole and there is no cardiac activity. Which length would suggest fetal demise?

   A. >2 cm
   B. >2 mm
   C. >5 cm
   D. >5 mm
   E. >10 mm

9. Trisomy 21 is associated with approximately what percentage of congenital heart defects?

   A. 100%
   B. 75%
   C. 50%
   D. 25%
   E. 10%

10. Which of these flow velocities across the ductus arteriosus is considered abnormal?

    A. >70 cm per second
    B. >84 cm per second
    C. >100 cm per second
    D. >120 cm per second
    E. >140 cm per second

11. You see two vessels posterior to the four-chamber heart view. What anomaly do you suspect?

    A. Tetralogy of Fallot
    B. Truncus arteriosus
    C. Right atrial isomerism
    D. Tricuspid atresia
    E. Interrupted inferior vena cava with azygos vein continuation

12. What is the risk that a congenital heart defect will recur when the mother is affected?

    A. No increased risk
    B. 2%–4%
    C. 5%–10%
    D. 10%–12%
    E. >15%

13. What is the reported sensitivity of the four-chamber heart view in detecting a congenital heart defect?

    A. 100%
    B. 85%–92%
    C. 50%–78%
    D. 10%–25%
    E. 40%–57%

14. Which of the following represents proper hand hygiene measures?

    A. Hand washing only if gloves are not worn during the examination.
    B. Hand washing or rubbing only if the technologist contacts body fluids or secretions during the ultrasound examination.
    C. Washing hands thoroughly with soap and water for 40–60 seconds after every examination.
    D. Rubbing hands completely with an alcohol-based product for 20–30 seconds until dry after every examination.
    E. Either C or D is acceptable.

15. Type II diabetes mellitus is defined as an increased Hgb A1C level of at least:

    A. 2.5%
    B. 3.5%
    C. 4.5%
    D. 6.5%
    E. 8.0%

16. Where is the pulmonic valve in relation to the aortic valve?

    A. Posterior and inferior
    B. Anterior and inferior
    C. Anterior and superior
    D. Posterior and superior
    E. At the same level

17. Absorption of energy from attenuation of the ultrasound beam is highest in what type of tissue/fluid?

    A. Bone
    B. Soft tissue
    C. Urine

D. Amniotic fluid

E. Blood

18. In addition to 3D real-time echocardiography, which of the following imaging modalities can be used to assess left ventricular function?

A. 4D sonography

B. B-mode sonography

C. Continuous-wave Doppler

D. A and C

E. A, B, and C

19. When is a fetal echocardiogram most commonly performed?

A. 16–18 weeks' gestation

B. 18–22 weeks' gestation

C. 22–26 weeks' gestation

D. 26–28 weeks' gestation

E. After 28 weeks' gestation

20. The majority of fetal cardiac output is through the:

A. Aorta

B. Ductus arteriosus

C. Left atrium

D. Right ventricle

E. None of the above

21. Which of these structures functions as the pacemaker of the heart?

A. Bundle of His

B. Sinoatrial node

C. Purkinje fibers

D. Atrioventricular node

E. Coronary sinus

22. Which of these statements about the E/A wave ratio of the mitral valve is TRUE?

A. It increases with advancing pregnancy.

B. It decreases with advancing pregnancy.

C. It fluctuates with advancing pregnancy.

D. It remains constant throughout the pregnancy.

E. None of the above.

23. A midline development field defect is thought to lead to which of the following conditions?

A. Ivemark syndrome

B. Polysplenia syndrome

C. Right atrial isomerism

D. Asplenia syndrome

E. All of the above

24. Polysplenia syndrome is also known as:

   A. Left atrial isomerism
   B. Bilateral left-sidedness
   C. Bilateral right-sidedness
   D. Shone syndrome
   E. Both A and B

25. Which syndrome is associated with a complex heart defect in 95%–100% of cases, may progress to bradycardia and complete heart block, and has a high mortality rate?

   A. Polysplenia syndrome
   B. Noonan syndrome
   C. Patau syndrome (trisomy 13)
   D. Ivemark syndrome
   E. Asplenia syndrome

26. What is the risk of a heart defect in cases of situs inversus with extreme levocardia?

   A. 2%
   B. 10%
   C. 25%
   D. 80%
   E. Nearly 100%

27. What does a fetal heart rate of 198 beats per minute with normal atrioventricular activation suggest?

   A. Normal fetal heart rate
   B. Supraventricular tachycardia
   C. Ventricular tachycardia
   D. Sinus tachycardia
   E. Premature ventricular contraction

28. To obtain the most precise image, where should the area of interest be focused?

   A. Divergent field
   B. Far field
   C. Near field
   D. Nyquist zone
   E. Frame path

29. Identify the most commonly recognized cardiac defect:

   A. Bicuspid aortic valve
   B. Pulmonic stenosis
   C. Atrioventricular septal defect
   D. Ventricular septal defect
   E. Atrial septal defect

30. Univentricular heart is classified by the presence or absence of:

    A. A moderator band
    B. Atrioventricular valves
    C. A rudimentary ventricular chamber
    D. A patent ductus arteriosus
    E. All of the above

31. Which fetal heart view best demonstrates the atrioventricular junction, including the valve leaflets and annulus?

    A. Apical four-chamber view
    B. Subcostal four-chamber view
    C. Apical five-chamber view
    D. Short-axis view
    E. A and B

32. When Doppler ultrasonography demonstrates pulsatile flow in the umbilical vein, it most likely represents:

    A. Volume overload
    B. Premature atrial contraction
    C. Normal Doppler flow pattern
    D. Congestive heart failure
    E. Both B and C

33. A massively enlarged right atrium is identified with an apically displaced tricuspid valve. What cardiac heart defect is most likely suggested by these findings?

    A. Tricuspid atresia
    B. Hypoplastic right heart syndrome
    C. Hypoplastic left heart syndrome
    D. Ebstein anomaly
    E. Uhl malformation

34. Which of the following maternal conditions is NOT an indication for a fetal echocardiographic exam?

    A. Maternal hyperthyroidism
    B. Maternal diabetes
    C. Maternal connective tissue disorder
    D. Maternal use of alcohol
    E. Maternal hyperphenylalaninemia (phenylketonuria)

35. What fetal anomaly, if found in isolation, does NOT warrant further evaluation with fetal echocardiography?

    A. Renal agenesis
    B. Dandy-Walker malformation
    C. Diaphragmatic hernia
    D. Omphalocele
    E. Gastroschisis

36. In the subcostal four-chamber view of the normal fetal heart, which cardiac structure is closest to the fetal spine?

    A. Mitral valve
    B. Left atrium
    C. Right atrium
    D. Right ventricle
    E. Left ventricle

37. Detecting multiple echoes within the right atrium, you know they can represent:

    A. Tricuspid valve leaflets
    B. Chiari network
    C. Foramen ovale flap
    D. Eustachian valve
    E. Both B and D

38. Disturbed bulboventricular loop development during the embryonic stage leads to:

    A. Asplenia
    B. Univentricular heart
    C. Polysplenia
    D. Atrioventricular septal defect
    E. Ventricular septal defect

39. The risk that a fetus will have an abnormal karyotype when a congenital heart defect is diagnosed on fetal ultrasound is:

    A. 100%
    B. 85%
    C. 50%
    D. 35%
    E. 15%

40. What leads to embryologic pulmonic stenosis?

    A. Abnormal intracardiac blood flow
    B. Abnormal targeted growth
    C. Cell death abnormality
    D. Tissue-migration abnormality
    E. Extracellular matrix abnormality

41. What is the most common type of cardiomyopathy?

    A. Congestive
    B. Hypertrophic
    C. Dilated
    D. Restrictive
    E. Both A and C

42. What is another name for *situs ambiguus*?

   A. Heterotaxy
   B. Levoposition
   C. Levorotation
   D. Dextrocardia
   E. Dextroposition

43. Which of these imaging modalities is used as an adjunct to M-mode for assessing fetal heart rate and rhythm?

   A. Spectral Doppler
   B. B-mode ultrasound
   C. Computed tomography
   D. 3D imaging
   E. Magnetic resonance imaging

44. The most common location of the ventricular septal defect with tetralogy of Fallot is:

   A. Apical
   B. Subpulmonic
   C. Subaortic
   D. Both A and C
   E. None of the above

45. Identify the most common type of pathologic tachycardia:

   A. Supraventricular tachycardia
   B. Atrial flutter
   C. Sinus tachycardia
   D. Ventricular tachycardia
   E. Premature atrial contraction

46. Which of the following is NOT true of shadowing artifacts?

   A. They appear as hypoechoic or anechoic.
   B. They represent multiple reflections of the same structure.
   C. They are located beneath the structure with abnormally high attenuation.
   D. They result from too much attenuation.
   E. They prevent visualization of true anatomy on the scan.

47. Which of the following syndromes is associated with truncus arteriosus?

   A. Noonan syndrome
   B. Williams syndrome
   C. DiGeorge syndrome
   D. Turner syndrome
   E. Down syndrome

48. Which sonographic modality displays a single B-mode line of site along a horizontal axis?

    A. M-mode
    B. B-color
    C. B-mode
    D. Pulsed-wave Doppler
    E. Spectral Doppler

49. Which term best describes postnatal circulation with d-transposition of the great arteries?

    A. Normal
    B. Series
    C. Parallel
    D. Reverse
    E. Restrictive

50. Which of the following maternal conditions is an indication for fetal echocardiography?

    A. In vitro fertilization
    B. Exposure to retinoids
    C. Exposure to lithium
    D. 22q11.2 deletion syndrome
    E. All of the above

51. Where does fetal gas exchange occur?

    A. In the umbilical vein
    B. In the umbilical artery
    C. In the placenta
    D. Through the ductus arteriosus
    E. In the fetal lungs

52. The Standard (Universal) Precautions are:

    A. Measures taken to prevent the transmission of blood-borne diseases
    B. Actions taken to create a barrier between you and potentially infected body fluids
    C. Methods of preventing transmission of blood-borne diseases
    D. Approaches to infection control
    E. All of the above

53. In utero, the normal patent ductal artery:

    A. Has a pulsatility index of 1.9–3.0
    B. Shunts blood from the pulmonary artery to aorta
    C. Shunts blood right to left
    D. May be constricted with indomethacin
    E. All of the above

54. What is the most common type of aortic stenosis?

    A. Subvalvular aortic stenosis
    B. Valvular aortic stenosis
    C. Aortic atresia
    D. Supravalvular aortic stenosis
    E. None of the above

55. Which of the following conditions can NOT be evaluated using the short-axis view of the ventricles?

    A. Interventricular septal defects
    B. Ventricular chamber size
    C. Fetal arrhythmias
    D. Ventricular free wall thickness
    E. The moderator band

56. What is the most common embryologic tissue-migration abnormality?

    A. Truncus arteriosus
    B. Tetralogy of Fallot
    C. D-transposition of the great arteries
    D. Double-outlet right ventricle
    E. Pulmonic stenosis with ventricular septal defect

57. The most common malformation in children born with cyanotic heart disease is:

    A. Truncus arteriosus
    B. Tetralogy of Fallot
    C. Double-outlet right ventricle
    D. D-transposition of the great arteries
    E. Univentricular heart

58. What is NOT seen on the routine four-chamber heart?

    A. Septal attachments of the tricuspid valve to the interventricular septum
    B. Foramen ovale flap bulging from right atrium to left atrium
    C. Aortic wall continuity with the interventricular septum
    D. Pulmonary veins being accepted into the left atrium
    E. Moderator band present in the right ventricle

59. What characterizes normal patent foramen ovale flow?

    A. Biphasic, 20–40 cm/sec
    B. Triphasic, 20–40 cm/sec
    C. Monophasic, 20–40 cm/sec
    D. Biphasic, 50–70 cm/sec
    E. Monophasic, 50–70 cm/sec

60. In the normal fetal heart, the most anterior structure is the:

    A. Pulmonary artery
    B. Right atrium

C. Aorta

D. Left ventricle

E. Right ventricle

61. What is the normal oxygen saturation of blood flowing into the fetus through the umbilical vein?

A. 65%

B. 85%

C. 45%

D. 55%

E. 75%

62. What is the incidence of heart defects among all live-born infants?

A. 20:1000 infants

B. 10:1000 infants

C. 4:1000 infants

D. 8:1000 infants

E. 1:1000 infants

63. In the fetus, maternal systemic lupus erythematosus may present with:

A. Sinus tachycardia

B. Premature atrial contractions

C. Complete heart block

D. Supraventricular tachycardia

E. Premature ventricular contractions

64. Which of these structures are visible in the long-axis view of the left heart?

A. Left atrium, mitral valve, and left ventricle

B. Right atrium, tricuspid valve, and papillary muscle

C. Left atrium, mitral valve, papillary muscle, left ventricle, and pulmonic valve

D. Left atrium, mitral valve, papillary muscle, right ventricle, and left ventricle

E. Papillary muscle, right ventricle, and pulmonic valve

65. Approximately when does the embryo's heart begin to beat?

A. 7–10 days

B. 12–14 days

C. 21–28 days

D. 28–38 days

E. 35–48 days

66. To evaluate for pulmonary valve insufficiency, the ideal fetal heart view is the:

A. Apical four-chamber view

B. Short-axis view of the great vessels

C. Apical long-axis view of the pulmonary artery

D. Subcostal four-chamber view

E. Both B and C

67. Your fetal patient has multiple tumors in the right and left ventricles of the heart and the mother has a history of tuberous sclerosis. What cardiac tumor do you suspect?

    A. Rhabdomyoma

    B. Teratoma

    C. Myxoma

    D. Fibroma

    E. Hemangioma

68. Maternal alcohol abuse is an indication for fetal echocardiography because it is associated with an increased risk for:

    A. Hypotelorism

    B. Turner syndrome

    C. Fetal alcohol syndrome

    D. Perinatal alcohol addiction

    E. Congenital heart defects

69. Atrial septal defects are commonly associated with the following syndrome:

    A. Turner syndrome

    B. Williams syndrome

    C. Holt-Oram syndrome

    D. Noonan syndrome

    E. Patau syndrome

70. The vessel in the fetal circulation that permits blood to bypass the liver is the:

    A. Umbilical artery

    B. Umbilical vein

    C. Ductus arteriosus

    D. Ductus venosus

    E. Portal vein

71. What is the most common type of ventricular septal defect?

    A. Inlet

    B. Membranous

    C. Trabecular

    D. Muscular

    E. Outlet

72. The structures that make up the ductal arch are the:

    A. Pulmonary artery, ductus arteriosus, and descending aorta

    B. Pulmonary artery, ascending aorta, and pulmonic valve

    C. Ductus arteriosus, ascending aorta, and descending aorta

    D. Ductus arteriosus, ascending aorta, and innominate artery

    E. Pulmonary artery, ductus arteriosus, and ascending aorta

73. In a normal fetal heart how many pulmonary veins drain into the left atrium?

    A. 1
    B. 2
    C. 3
    D. 4
    E. 5

74. Which modality transmits the greatest amount of energy into the fetus?

    A. Pulsed-wave Doppler
    B. 2D imaging
    C. Power Doppler
    D. Color Doppler
    E. M-mode

75. The syndrome associated with an interrupted inferior vena cava and an azygos vein continuation is:

    A. Left atrial isomerism
    B. Ivemark syndrome
    C. Asplenia syndrome
    D. Polysplenia syndrome
    E. Both A and D

76. A fetus whose routine 35-week ultrasound reveals supraventricular tachycardia develops hydrops and has poor fetal testing. What is the recommended treatment?

    A. Immediate delivery
    B. Another ultrasound exam in one week
    C. Maternal digoxin therapy
    D. Percutaneous umbilical cord blood sampling procedure
    E. No treatment

77. Which of the following vessels allows blood flow to bypass the fetal lungs?

    A. Aorta
    B. Ductus arteriosus
    C. Superior vena cava
    D. Left pulmonary artery
    E. Ductus venosus

78. How many cusps does the normal aortic valve have?

    A. 2 cusps
    B. 3 cusps
    C. 4 cusps
    D. 5 cusps
    E. 6 cusps

79. Ultrasound energy causes a rise in temperature in the tissues through which it travels. Which of the following is NOT a significant temperature increase?
    A. <1 degree Celsius
    B. <1.5 degrees Celsius
    C. <2.0 degrees Celsius
    D. <2.2 degrees Celsius
    E. No rise in temperature is safe.

80. Which of the following statements about the normal mitral valve is TRUE?
    A. It is continuous with the posterior wall of the aorta.
    B. It has anterior, posterior, and septal leaflets.
    C. It is attached more apically than the tricuspid leaflets.
    D. Both B and C.
    E. All of the above.

81. A persistent left superior vena cava is often associated with:
    A. Ostium primum atrial septal defect
    B. Coronary sinus atrial septal defect
    C. Sinus venosus atrial septal defect
    D. Ostium secundum atrial septal defect
    E. Atrioventricular septal defect

82. When is the best time to measure nuchal translucency?
    A. 8–10 weeks' gestation
    B. 11–14 weeks' gestation
    C. 14–18 weeks' gestation
    D. 18–23 weeks' gestation
    E. 24–26 weeks' gestation

83. A fetus has an atrial heart rate of 300–500 beats per minute with varying ventricular response. What do you suspect?
    A. Atrial bigeminy
    B. Ventricular tachycardia
    C. Sinus tachycardia
    D. Atrial flutter
    E. Premature atrial contractions

84. To evaluate the number of aortic cusps, the best view is the:
    A. Short-axis view of the great vessels
    B. Subcostal four-chamber view
    C. Long-axis view of the pulmonary artery
    D. Apical four-chamber view
    E. Long-axis view of the aorta

85. Which cardiac anomaly is most commonly associated with hypoplastic left heart syndrome?

    A. Endocardial fibroelastosis
    B. Interrupted aortic arch
    C. Pulmonic stenosis
    D. Tachycardia
    E. Coarctation of the aorta

86. The most common cardiac cause of death in the early neonate is:

    A. Complete heart block
    B. Hypoplastic left heart syndrome
    C. Patent ductus arteriosus
    D. Atrial septal defect
    E. Hypoplastic right heart syndrome

87. What is the most commonly seen teratogenic heart lesion in the fetus?

    A. Tetralogy of Fallot
    B. Atrial septal defect
    C. Truncus arteriosus
    D. Ventricular septal defect
    E. Atrioventricular septal defect

88. What sonographic view should be obtained to diagnose a right-sided aortic arch?

    A. Three-vessel view
    B. Long-axis view of the aorta
    C. Apical four-chamber view
    D. Subcostal four-chamber view
    E. Short-axis view of the great arteries

89. What is the first step in any fetal echocardiographic exam?

    A. Identify the stomach location
    B. Establish fetal position
    C. Identify the arch sidedness
    D. Establish sex of the baby
    E. Identify the ventricles

90. In d-transposition of the great arteries, the aorta:

    A. Is connected to the left ventricle
    B. Is connected to the right ventricle
    C. Is connected to the pulmonary artery
    D. Is connected to the left atrium
    E. Overrides a ventricular septal defect

91. What percentage of the thoracic cavity area does the normal fetal heart occupy?

    A. 50%
    B. ≧75%
    C. 15%
    D. ≦33%
    E. 25%

92. Identify the vessels in the three-vessel view, listed in order from the vessel with the largest diameter to the vessel with the smallest diameter in the normal thorax:

    A. Pulmonary artery > superior vena cava > aorta
    B. Aorta > pulmonary artery > superior vena cava
    C. Pulmonary artery > aorta > superior vena cava
    D. Superior vena cava > aorta > pulmonary artery
    E. Aorta > superior vena cava > pulmonary artery

93. In Ebstein anomaly, which leaflet has a sail-like appearance?

    A. Posterior leaflet of tricuspid valve
    B. Anterior leaflet of tricuspid valve
    C. Septal leaflet of mitral valve
    D. Both A and B
    E. All of the above

94. Which of these congenital heart defects is caused by the failure of the endocardial cushions to fuse properly?

    A. Atrial septal defect
    B. Univentricular heart
    C. Ventricular septal defect
    D. Hypoplastic left heart syndrome
    E. Atrioventricular septal defect

95. Why is nonimmune fetal hydrops an indication for fetal echocardiography?

    A. It suggests the presence of structural heart defects.
    B. It indicates the presence of alloimmune hemolytic disease.
    C. It may indicate fetal cardiac dysrhythmias.
    D. It suggests complications from Rh isoimmunization.
    E. A and C.

96. What is the most common fetal cardiac finding associated with diabetic mothers?

    A. Double-outlet right ventricle
    B. Double-outlet left ventricle
    C. Hypertrophic cardiomyopathy
    D. Truncus arteriosus
    E. Both A and D

97. In what percentage of cases is duodenal atresia associated with a congenital heart defect?

    A. 78.0%
    B. 52.0%
    C. 5.2%
    D. 25.4%
    E. 17.1%

98. Which of the following conditions would, if it were part of the family history, warrant a fetal echocardiography exam?

    A. DiGeorge syndrome
    B. Holt-Oram syndrome
    C. Marfan syndrome
    D. A and B only
    E. All of the above

99. In coarctation of the aorta, the aortic narrowing almost always occurs at what level?

    A. Between the left common carotid artery and the subclavian artery
    B. Between the left subclavian artery and the ductus arteriosus
    C. Between the innominate artery and the left common carotid artery
    D. Distal to the ductal arch
    E. Between the ascending aorta and the innominate artery

100. Most blood flow entering the right atrium shunts to the left atrium through the:

    A. Pulmonary artery
    B. Pulmonary veins
    C. Patent foramen ovale
    D. Coronary sinus
    E. Sinus venosus

101. Identify the most common type of double-outlet right ventricle:

    A. Double-outlet right ventricle with a doubly committed ventricular septal defect (VSD)
    B. Double-outlet right ventricle with a subpulmonic VSD
    C. Double-outlet right ventricle with a remote VSD
    D. Double-outlet right ventricle with a subaortic VSD
    E. Double-outlet right ventricle with no VSD

102. Which of the following cardiac lesions has a hemodynamic communication between the right and left ventricles?

    A. Septum primum atrial septal defect
    B. Patent foramen ovale
    C. Ventricular septal defect
    D. Semilunar valve
    E. Septum secundum atrial septal defect

103. When the apex of the fetal heart is pointing to the fetal left chest with the axis at 45 degrees, what is this termed?

    A. Mesocardia
    B. Dextrocardia
    C. Levocardia
    D. Levorotated
    E. Dextroposition

104. In what percentage of cases is polysplenia associated with other cardiac anomalies?

    A. 8%–10%
    B. 25%–45%
    C. 45%–65%
    D. 75%–80%
    E. 90%–95%

105. Which statement accurately defines a heart rhythm with an early atrial beat that is not followed by a ventricular beat?

    A. Premature atrial contraction
    B. Supraventricular tachycardia
    C. Complete atrioventricular block
    D. Blocked premature atrial contraction
    E. Partial atrioventricular block

106. What function is used to eliminate low-frequency noise and artifactual clutter caused by the movement of vessel walls?

    A. Wall filter
    B. Time gain compensation
    C. Edge enhancement
    D. Pulse inversion
    E. Baseline

107. What are the advantages of power Doppler compared to color Doppler?

    A. Power Doppler is useful in slow-flow velocity states.
    B. Power Doppler is less dependent on the angle of incidence.
    C. Power Doppler is less dependent on direction of blood flow.
    D. Power Doppler is not subject to aliasing.
    E. All of the above are benefits.

108. If a fetus has fetal alcohol syndrome, the risk of cardiac anomaly is:

    A. 40%–50%
    B. 5%–10%
    C. 25%–30%
    D. 2%–4%
    E. No increased risk

109. In a fetus with double-outlet right ventricle, what is the most common location for a ventricular septal defect?

    A. Doubly committed
    B. Subaortic
    C. Subpulmonary
    D. Remote
    E. Both B and C

110. What is the relationship of the great arteries with tricuspid atresia?

    A. Normal
    B. D-transposition (complete)
    C. L-transposition (corrected)
    D. Divided equally
    E. Undifferentiated

111. What term describes the location where the sound beam reaches its narrowest diameter during ultrasound interrogation?

    A. Near field
    B. Far field
    C. Bandwidth
    D. Focal zone
    E. Frame path

112. Atrioventricular septal defect with tetralogy of Fallot is associated with:

    A. Patau syndrome (trisomy 13)
    B. Down syndrome (trisomy 21)
    C. Edwards syndrome (trisomy 18)
    D. Asplenia syndrome
    E. Polysplenia syndrome

113. Of the four classic features of tetralogy of Fallot, which is generally NOT seen in utero?

    A. Right ventricular hypertrophy
    B. Ventricular septal defect
    C. Overriding aorta
    D. Pulmonic stenosis
    E. All of the above are commonly seen in utero.

114. What adjustment can you make to visualize flow in vessels with low flow states such as the pulmonary veins?

    A. Increase scale.
    B. Decrease the color gain.
    C. Decrease the pulse repetition frequency.
    D. Adjust overall gain.
    E. All of the above.

115. The atrial-to-ventricular ratio in a normal fetus should be:

    A. 1:1
    B. 1:2
    C. 1:3
    D. 2:1
    E. 3:1

116. In a fetus, the most common cardiac tumor is:

    A. Hemangioma
    B. Rhabdomyoma
    C. Myoxoma
    D. Teratoma
    E. Fibroma

117. What is the most common cardiac venous anomaly?

    A. Azygos vein continuation
    B. Absent ductus venosus
    C. Persistent left superior vena cava
    D. Umbilical vein aneurysm
    E. Interrupted inferior vena cava

118. What artifact is caused by two strong reflectors with a large surface area, is displayed in the near field, and has multiple, equally spaced echoes extending into the far field?

    A. Bandwidth artifact
    B. Side-lobe artifact
    C. Reverberation artifact
    D. Mirror-image artifact
    E. Speckle artifact

119. The most common form of interrupted aortic arch is:

    A. Type I
    B. Type II
    C. Type A
    D. Type B
    E. Type C

120. All of the following are considered to be cardiac tumors EXCEPT:

    A. Echogenic foci
    B. Rhabdomyoma
    C. Fibroma
    D. Myxoma
    E. Hemangioma

PART 10

ARDMS Exam Content Outline Tasks Cross-Referenced to Mock Exam Questions

Note: *For your convenience, the mock exam questions in* Fetal Echocardiography Review *are arranged below according to the task-related topics and subtopics of the ARDMS exam content outline (see www.ardms.org). After each ARDMS task is a list of the question numbers from this mock exam that pertain to that task.*

Anatomy & Physiology—25%

Normal anatomy and physiology

Evaluate aortic arch: 1, 2, 3, 4, 5, 6, 7, 65, 164, 202.

Evaluate cardiac chambers: 8, 9, 10, 11, 12, 13, 14, 16, 17, 18, 20, 21, 23, 33, 34, 35, 36, 37, 73, 370.

Evaluate cardiac septa and related structures (e.g., foramen ovale): 15, 17, 25, 26, 27, 83, 368, 395, 401.

Evaluate cardiac valves: 19, 22, 28, 29, 30, 31, 32, 69, 145, 379, 400.

Evaluate coronary vessels: 36, 37, 38, 39, 40, 41, 42, 43.

Evaluate ductal arch: 44, 45, 81, 387, 388.

Evaluate fetal anatomic structures related to the abdomen/pelvis (e.g., hepatic veins, stomach. bladder, spleen, etc.): 46, 47, 48, 71, 263.

Evaluate fetal anatomic structures related to the chest/thorax (e.g., lungs, esophagus, trachea, etc.): 49, 50, 51, 63, 153, 370.

Evaluate fetus for normal cardiac axis, cardiac position, and abdominal situs: 52, 53, 54, 55, 56, 57.

Evaluate pulmonary vessels (i.e., pulmonary arteries, pulmonary veins): 1, 7, 24, 43, 44, 58, 59, 60, 61, 62, 64, 66, 67, 68, 70, 81, 90, 96, 183, 186, 372, 375, 380.

Evaluate systemic vessels: 4, 27, 36, 44, 45, 71, 72, 79, 81, 82, 83, 85, 88, 89, 90, 186, 252, 375, 377, 385, 387, 389.

Evaluate tissues composing the heart: 10, 11, 13, 73, 74, 97, 365.

Perfusion and function

Evaluate for normal cardiac rhythms: 74, 75, 76, 77, 78, 108.

Evaluate for normal fetal circulation: 27, 45, 72, 79, 80, 81, 82, 83, 84, 85, 86, 87, 88, 89, 90.

Organ development

Assess for normal embryologic development: 74, 78, 91, 92, 93, 94, 95, 96, 97, 98, 99, 100, 101, 102, 303, 347.

Perform various fetal echocardiographic examinations during appropriate time intervals: 78, 103, 104, 466.

Pathology—20%

Abnormal perfusion and function

Assess for signs of fetal distress in response to placental or maternal injury/insult: 105, 106, 110, 210, 325, 341, 342, 402, 403, 453.

Evaluate for the presence of fetal cardiomyopathies: 107, 108, 109, 110, 111, 112, 113, 117, 333, 473.

Evaluate for the presence of fetal dysrhythmias: 105, 114, 115, 116, 117, 118, 119, 120, 121, 122, 123, 124, 125, 126, 127, 276, 320, 334, 345, 356, 390, 391, 397, 398, 470.

Evaluate the aortic valve: 29, 128, 129, 130, 132, 169, 212, 337.

Evaluate the mitral valve: 28, 75, 130, 131, 212, 213, 288.

Evaluate the pulmonary valve: 128, 132, 133, 134, 135, 136, 233, 235, 243, 245, 275.

Evaluate the tricuspid valve: 137, 138, 139, 140, 141, 142, 143, 144, 145, 232, 236, 244.

Congenital anomalies

Evaluate for cardiac malpositioning (e.g., mesocardia, levoposition, ambiguus, inversus, etc.): 146, 147, 148, 149, 150, 151, 152, 153, 272, 324.

Evaluate for congenital cardiac septal defects: 154, 155, 156, 157, 158, 159, 160, 161, 162, 163, 164, 165, 166, 167, 168, 169, 170, 171, 172, 175, 199, 226, 231, 242, 245, 247, 248, 254, 256, 257, 271, 304, 401.

Evaluate for conotruncal abnormalities: 128, 136, 144, 160, 164, 165, 166, 168, 171, 173, 174, 175, 176, 177, 178, 179, 180, 181, 182, 183, 184, 185, 186, 187, 188, 189, 190, 191, 192, 193, 194, 195, 196, 197, 198, 199, 201, 202, 203, 206, 211, 217, 221, 235, 237, 238, 239, 240, 241, 243, 249, 277, 286, 311, 327, 328, 361, 362, 467.

Evaluate for left-sided cardiac anomalies: 128, 129, 130, 160, 164, 169, 171, 173, 199, 200, 201, 202, 203, 204, 205, 206, 207, 208, 209, 210, 211, 212, 213, 214, 215, 216, 217, 218, 219, 220, 221, 222, 240, 242, 247, 248, 274, 283, 359.

Evaluate for pulmonary venous anomalies: 168, 223, 224, 225, 226, 227, 228, 229, 230, 231.

Evaluate for right-sided cardiac anomalies: 128, 135, 136, 142, 145, 165, 171, 173, 199, 216, 218, 219, 232, 233, 234, 235, 236, 237, 238, 239, 240, 241, 242, 243, 244, 245, 246, 247, 248, 249, 250, 251, 275.

Evaluate for systemic venous anomalies: 172, 252, 253, 254, 255, 256, 257, 258, 259, 260, 261, 262, 263, 264, 279.

Evaluate for the presence of congenital cardiac masses: 265, 266, 267, 268, 269, 306.

Evaluate the fetus for sonographic signs related to various genetic syndromes (e.g., Down, Noonan, Turner, etc.): 115, 253, 264, 270, 271, 272, 273, 274, 275, 276, 277, 278, 279, 280, 281, 282, 283, 284, 285, 286, 287, 288, 289, 290, 291, 292, 293, 294, 307, 308, 309, 310, 311, 469.

Patient Care—5%

Infection control

Maintain infection control: 296, 297, 298, 299.

Practice Universal Precautions: 295, 300, 301.

Integration of Data—15%

Incorporate outside data (Clinical assessment, Health & Physical [H&P], Lab values)

Assess indications for performing a fetal echocardiogram: 302, 303, 304, 317, 326, 348, 351.

Obtain pertinent medical history of patient: 105, 110, 112, 246, 305, 306, 326, 327, 328, 329, 330, 337, 340, 341, 345.

Use chromosomal anomalies or genetic syndromes as exam indicators: 110, 307, 308, 309, 310, 311, 348, 350.

Use family history as exam indicator: 312, 313, 314, 315, 316.

Use fetal clinical signs and symptoms to guide the echocardiogram: 105, 317, 318, 319, 345, 472.

Use fetal dysrhythmias as exam indicators: 317, 320, 329, 345, 470, 471, 472.

Use fetal extracardiac malformations as exam indicators: 321, 322, 323, 324.

Use hydrops as exam indicator: 106, 318, 325, 402, 470, 472, 474.

Use maternal diseases as exam indicators: 105, 110, 112, 305, 306, 326, 327, 328, 329, 330, 331, 332, 333, 334, 335, 336, 337, 338.

Use maternal drug exposure as exam indicator: 246, 326, 339, 340, 341, 342, 343, 344, 345, 346, 347, 348.

Use suspected cardiac abnormality on an outside scan as exam indicator: 319, 336, 349, 350, 351, 352.

Use thickened nuchal translucency as exam indicator: 294, 319, 352, 353, 354.

Reporting results

Compare echocardiographic results to other imaging modalities: 355, 356, 357, 358, 359, 393, 439, 450, 451.

Protocols—10%

Clinical standards and guidelines

Demonstrate the cardiac five-chamber view: 360, 361.

Demonstrate the four-chamber views (i.e., apical, subcostal): 14, 15, 16, 59, 362, 363, 364, 365, 366, 367, 368, 369, 370, 395.

Demonstrate the long-axis views (i.e., aorta, pulmonary artery): 4, 5, 6, 7, 32, 33, 34, 35, 133, 361, 369, 371, 372, 373, 374, 376.

Demonstrate the orientation of the great vessels using various cardiac views: 31, 373, 375, 376, 377, 378, 379.

Demonstrate the pulmonary vein and branches views: 24, 59, 61, 369, 380.

Demonstrate the short-axis views (i.e., ventricles, great vessels): 67, 68, 69, 70, 133, 362, 369, 381, 382, 383, 384, 395.

Demonstrate the three-vessel view: 41, 42, 43, 49, 63, 64, 65, 66, 375, 385, 386.

Demonstrate the various views of the arches (i.e., aortic, ductal): 387, 388.

Demonstrate the vena caval views: 36, 41, 71, 389.

Use Doppler to evaluate fetal heart rate: 356, 390, 391.

Use M-mode to evaluate fetal heart rate: 108, 392, 393, 394, 395, 396, 397, 398.

Measurement techniques

Perform fetal cardiac biometry measurements to assess visualized cardiac structures (e.g., valve annuli, aortic and ductal arches, chamber sizes, etc.): 2, 28, 32, 75, 395, 399, 400, 401.

Perform various gray-scale measurements to assess visualized cardiac structures: 17, 18, 19, 20, 21, 22, 23, 24, 25, 370, 395.

Perform various gray-scale measurements to assess visualized pathology: 108, 132, 383, 399, 401, 402, 403.

Physics & Instrumentation—20%

Imaging instruments

Adjust console settings to achieve optimal imaging display: 404, 405, 406, 407, 408, 409, 410.

Perform quality assurance checks on the equipment: 411, 412, 413, 414, 415, 416.

Select the proper transducer: 404, 416, 417, 418.

Artifacts

Modify the console settings based on color Doppler artifacts: 419, 420, 436.

Modify the console settings based on gray-scale artifacts: 421, 422, 423, 424, 425, 426, 427, 428, 429, 430.

Modify the console settings based on spectral Doppler artifacts: 420, 431, 432, 433, 434, 435, 436, 437.

Hemodynamics

Use color Doppler to assess blood flow: 438, 439, 440, 441, 442, 443, 444, 445, 446.

Use power Doppler to assess blood flow: 447, 448, 449, 450.

Use pulsed-wave Doppler to assess blood flow: 75, 76, 131, 451, 452, 453, 454, 455, 456, 457, 458, 459, 460, 461, 462, 463.

Other—5%

Managing medical emergencies

Assist patient experiencing a vasovagal response: 464, 465.

Inform the supervising physician of findings of an emergent nature (e.g., no fetal tone, hydrops, etc.): 106, 325, 342, 466, 467, 468, 469, 470, 471, 472, 473, 474, 475.